Endorsements

"What I appreciate most about Randy is that he is interested in my overall health including my mental, spiritual, and social well-being in addition to my physical health. He challenges me to think deeper on a multitude of issues that ultimately have served to improve my overall outlook on life and my health."

Jay Easaw MD, PHD, FRCP(C)

"No matter how many times I've been knocked down by life, Randy has always helped me get back on my feet and moving again. He has done extensive volunteer work for decades, both at the YMCA and in areas that are not just to do with physical wellness, but also mental health."

Tema Frank
Author "People Shock"

"Randy has a laser focus when it comes to fitness. While he teaches techniques he also educates his clients, not using the "lingo" but in a way that they understand the role that nutrition and exercise play in physical fitness and wellness. As a good listener, he helps his clients clarify their goals."

Lois Browne PHD

LIFE LESSONS FROM THE GYM

THE MENTAL GAME OF TRANSFORMATION

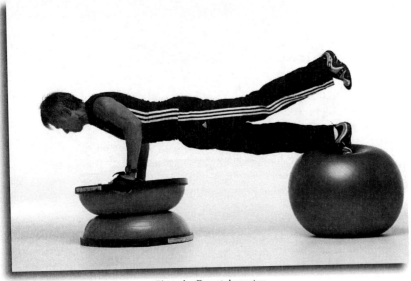

Photo by Ernest Augustus

Randy "Bumpa" Lee

nowgogetpumped!!!LIFE LESSONS FROM THE GYM
The Mental Game of TransformationThe 20.20.30.30 Method

© 2019 R.T. Lee & Associates
First Edition, 2020

Published by Randy "Bumpa" Lee, Edmonton, Canada

Photographs on front and back cover taken by Ernest Augustus

ISBN 0-978-1-99929-500-4

Publication assistance and digital printing in Canada by

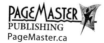

PUBLISHING
PageMaster.ca

Dedication

This book is lovingly dedicated to my beautiful wife Kim Franklin (TheKim) see Chapter 75... or Mummatinnie (as our granddaughter named her many years ago), the most loving, supportive, encouraging and accepting person in my world. Please don't tell her this, but she's very easy going, unlike me, which has taught me many ways to create more balance in my life.

Without her this book would not be in your hands, believe me. I love her to bits! She's my pickleball partner band bud best friend angel and she rocks my world!

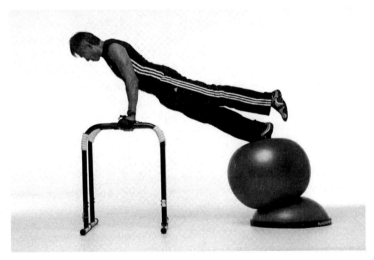

Photo by Ernest Augustus

Contents

20% Recovery 189

The Plan Man! 203

Conclusion 205

Two Thumbs Up 206

Bonus Bumpa Stickers 208

INTRODUCTION – Our Deal

I wrote this book to give you hope! My mission is to empower you to make personal changes in your life that will lead to a feeling of accomplishment... happiness... fulfillment and joy. Then you will be positioned to realize your full potential and to make your greatest contribution to the world. That's my vision!

A few years ago I was at a party having a great discussion with a 95 year old gal who was as sharp as a tack and holding her own very nicely in a playful verbal joust with me. I remember asking her what she thought of the current world situation. With a look of disgust, she turned to me and stared me straight in the eyes and said, "Randy, the whole world has gone to hell in a hand basket! Human kind is devolving!"

Now she could be right. Without sounding preachy... my view of the world is that we're in trouble.

Companies and people are doing things to each other that fly directly in the face of the First Law of the Universe: the Law of Cause and Effect - what you put out is what you get back.

People are lost, broken and stuck. There is way too much despair, anxiety, self-doubt, stress, frustration and depression. I think the main reason is that people lack joy and fulfillment in their lives. Not having these two critical basic components leads to, at best giving up and at worst, hostility.

If people continue to wander aimlessly, feeling helpless and unfulfilled, there will be even more hostility and discord.

I also believe that if people were able to find a way to do something really meaningful for themselves, life changing, and succeed at it, they would become unstuck, feel more accomplished and positive about themselves and everything around them, leading to even more successes. They could find peace, happiness, and their passion in life which would empower them to make their contribution. The legacy only they can bestow.

Then if they were to share their successes with two other people (remember the old commercial... "and they told two people... and they told two people"... and so on?) that we could, in fact, help other people do something really positive for themselves and then for our entire planet!

A very rewarding accomplishment that most people desire and would love to achieve is a physical transformation... usually to lose body fat and to look, feel and perform better. The challenge is that for various reasons, it seems out of reach for most people.

I firmly believe that if people want to change their lives, they should begin one step at a time.

Change begins with you! Start with a physical transformation. This change will increase self-esteem and confidence, and develop fantastic habits and skills. Then transfer all the skills you've learned to create a transformation in all the other areas of your life... physical, mental, spiritual, business, and relationships.

Since 1974 my ultimate passions have been health, fitness, nutrition and motivation, and now, using what I've learned, I sincerely want to help you change your LIFE!

I am going to show you, through the conversations and techniques in this book, how to transform your body into YOUR VERY BEST BODY, how to transform yourself into YOUR VERY BEST SELF!

Please... MAKE NO MISTAKE! The invaluable tools and skills that you will learn in this book will not only transform your body and serve you all the rest of your days, but they are highly transferable to every aspect of your life.

There is a reason that when Bill Phillips held his Body for Life Transformation Contest in 1997, he required not just a great transformation, but a 400 word essay explaining the trials and tribulations that contestants had to overcome in order to achieve their great results. The same "challenges" that may be preventing you from being successful in certain areas of your life are probably the same ones preventing you from being as healthy and as fit as you would like. Procrastination, lack of focus, lack of determination, and lack of knowledge... all are deterrents to success in any endeavor. Conquering them while creating a new body will lead to success in life, IF the skills learned are transferred.

I'm going to say this again in a slightly different way, because THIS, is a take home message!

If you don't have the body that you would like, in most cases the culprits that hold you back are the very same ones that are impeding the achievement of other goals in your life. Think about it. Is it a lack of motivation, procrastination, lack of persistence, ignorance, or perhaps self-sabotage that is preventing you from becoming your best self?

Interestingly, the very same techniques to acquire that hot bod are the exact same concepts, strategies and tools that will create success in your work life, your family life, your financial life, your social life, your spiritual life, and every other aspect of your life.

How to Use This Book

The chapters in this book don't have to be read in any particular order. Choose one of the four sections of interest to you. Each contains conversations that have taken place over the years between me and various clients and members. A conversation represents a chapter and addresses a key aspect of the transformation process, and will end with a **"Transferable Life Skill"**, a lesson that can be applied to your business, your relationships, everything that you would like to succeed at.

This makes it very easy to read the book in chunks as you have time.

Now this book may be a simple quick read but please, be not deceived. The journey is simple... but it's not always easy. If it was easy, everyone would be doing it, and everyone would look like a fitness model and everyone would be successful in life! Once you learn the principles, the strategies and the techniques, your life transformation will be astounding!

It would be very wise to read each conversation and transferable life skill, then STOP. Examine your life and/or business and apply the particular skill to an area that could benefit by the strategy or technique, perhaps an area where you have become "stuck". Contemplate and consider the message for the entire day in all that you do and then go on to the next chapter/conversation.

I believe that with every book, every movie, every presentation, the goal is to find at least one great take home message that can change your life for the better. This book contains many such messages.

My sincere hope for you is that you will read this book and use the strategies and techniques to transform your "physical" body first. And through that process, transfer the skills that you have learned to every other important area of your life... making you the very best version of yourself that is possible.

It doesn't stop there though. **Here's our deal.** People will most assuredly compliment you on your great transformation and ask you how you did it. When you hear those well-deserved words, "Wow, you're looking great, everything in your life has come together so nicely!" I want to encourage you to help two other people gain the same success that you have achieved, using the same ideas. You "GET TO" pay it forward!

For if you believe as I do, that the only way to reach fulfillment and true joy in this world is to help others... then when you do transform, first your body, then your life, and share your journey with others, this is the way we can all do our part to create a better planet! People will be less depressed, less lethargic, and less hostile. They will have more self-respect and satisfaction. They will be happier, more confident, more accomplished, more fulfilled, and as a result, more productive and more giving. They will, in fact, become much more capable of fulfilling their destiny and making their unique contribution.

My history will explain my dream.

My story starts out in Edmonton, Alberta, Canada in the spring of 1953. I was the first of three children born to a 2nd generation poor Chinese family.

As far back as I can remember, my mom was always trying to lose weight. She was either on the Cabbage Soup Diet, the Grapefruit Diet, the Atkins Diet, the Stillman Diet, the Scarsdale Diet, the Beverly Hills Diet or any one of the other temporary "quick fixes" of the day... or she was jumping up & down in front of the TV with some fitness guru.

Mom never really succeeded. She would always give up too soon and fall for the next new fad to come down the pipe. She made health and fitness a lifestyle alright... a lifestyle of never ending searches for the silver bullet.

People like my mom are struggling to find something they can believe, something that works, something satisfying, some accomplishment. If only they had the information, the strategies, the techniques and the confidence to see it through.

Your search will stop here. You will create a lifestyle of healthy eating and functional fitness using proven strategies that have taken over 45 years to compile.

The 30.30.20.20 Method

It has been said by many "experts" that fitness is 80 per cent nutrition and 20 per cent exercise. I don't believe that's true! If the equation is 80/20 then we're ignoring critical reasons why so few people get the results they seek.

My experience and observations tell me the equation is 30 per cent Psychological, 30 per cent Nutrition, 20 per cent Exercise, and 20 per cent Recovery. We cannot ignore the other two crucial components, recovery and psychological.

If there is no recovery component, the influence of certain hormones is affected and a multitude of challenges arise... tissue repair, energy issues and food cravings being but a few.

If there wasn't a psychological component, then motivational issues and self-sabotage wouldn't play such a huge part for so many people.

That's why this method is called 30.30.20.20. Part 1 of the book will present conversations on the Psychological aspect of transformation, Part 2 will be on Nutrition, Part 3 on Exercise and Part 4 on Recovery.

Upon leaving my psychology studies at university to take a summer job with a world-wide fitness chain, my advancement was meteoric, making me the youngest club manager at 21 years old in the entire organization. It would lead me on a fascinating lifelong adventure into the world of health and fitness that has uncovered what most people have not yet discovered... that it's really a mental journey. It's composed of transferable skills and it must be shared.

The scene was set because since that time I have always had a gym (playground) in my home and trained six days per week. I "experiment" regularly with nutrition and different exercise modalities for fun and education. A test drive, so to speak, to see what works and what doesn't.

After taking the incredible XOCES personal development seminar with Bob Proctor in 1975 my dream was born. My heart told me that I needed to share information with people to help them become all they could be. My thought processes, my belief system, my life, changed dramatically and I embarked on a life long journey to learn as much as I possibly could about human motivation. I took courses and attended seminars, all the while collecting hundreds of books and tapes, and spending every spare moment in self-discovery.

This led my fitness career path on a "sabbatical" into another "adventure". I became a Success Coach and VP of Operations for a division of Success Motivation Institute, where I conducted courses on goal setting, attitude, time management, environment, motivation and effective communication.

Once I retired, I volunteered with various organizations, including over twenty years as a counsellor & co-facilitator for men's groups through the City of Edmonton, and at the YMCA as an Individual Strength and Conditioning coach which continues to this day.

Many of my clients and members, who I've gleefully terrorized over the years, have become my very close friends over time so I have not only changed their names, but in some cases I have changed their genders to protect the innocent... and the not so innocent.

I know that together, we can make a difference. We can change our planet for the better!

Let's go... get unstuck... and change some lives... starting with yours!

nowgogetpumped!!!

PART 1

30% Psychological
The Mental Game

In the effort to transform your bod, exercise and nutrition are key elements. But they're not enough. I had to "quantify" the psychological factor... 30%. Perhaps it should be a higher percentage because if a person doesn't get this one right, all is for naught. If a person DOES nail the mental game, EVERYTHING becomes infinitely easier, and results in any endeavor are practically guaranteed! Attitude is EVERYTHING!

Why do people not exercise or eat well? Heck, they would never consider leaving the house each morning without brushing their teeth. But skipping exercise is par for the course.

This is a question that has really eluded me and caused me great frustration. No... the correct word is heartbreak. Often I want results for people more than they want it for themselves.

I just didn't get it! I would work with people who loved to exercise, resigned themselves to exercise, or reluctantly forced themselves to exercise. The same with nutrition. They loved to eat in a healthy manner, resigned themselves to it, or forced themselves.

The fact that they were training with me was a huge step in the right direction, although a few would admit that they would never walk into a playground if I weren't with them. Some of them didn't. They would train reluctantly when I was with them but when they were on their own to do their follow up sessions, they would conveniently find other things to do.

Likewise with nutrition. Armed with my certifications in Nutrition and Weight Loss, as well as Sports Nutrition, I would attempt to educate and encourage my members and clients to eat in a manner that would ensure that they achieved their goals.

Trainers have a saying; "You can't out train a bad diet!"

I have the FUNtabulous opportunity to train some of the most intelligent people on the planet who you would expect to "get it". But even some of them won't adhere to the program consistently. I've suggested reasons to make their health a priority; loved ones, quality of life, longevity, increased mental and physical function, disease prevention, weight control, and even to look fit and strong. It can be lost on the best of them.

Unfortunately, sometimes a person has to have an "event" to wake them up to the importance of a good health program. Hopefully that "event" would be witnessing another's health issue, and not experiencing their own. Or it has been said that, at some point, you just gotta get "sick and tired of being sick and tired"!

Napoleon Hill says that desire for any goal needs to be a burning desire like the one required to pull your head from a bucket of water when someone else is holding it submerged with both hands.

Solomon says that people don't do what they should do for three reasons. Either they're ignorant (they don't know the benefits). They're self-centered (they think they know better... it won't happen to them, or the research is bad, etc.). Or... they're just irresponsible. Yikes. How do I get around that one? Helping an adult become responsible and grow up is probably out of my scope of practice!

Jim Rohn said, "If you should... and you could... but you don't... and you won't... you messed up!" So very many people have messed up their lives by not doing what they should and could.

One of our dear friends has broken numerous bones by falling or simply by walking, yet she insists on getting her exercise by walking. She won't do any bone strengthening resistance training, or core training to prevent falling in the first place. That's messed up!

I hope that the conversations regarding the crucial psychological aspect that follow will answer some questions, and enlighten and motivate you to become your very best self!

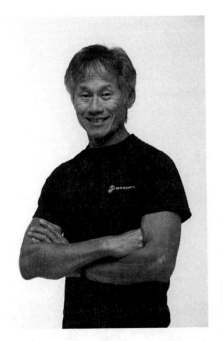 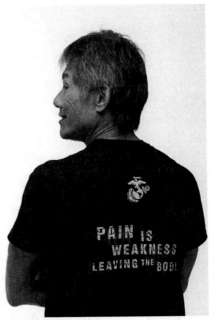

The Pullup T-shirt
Photos by Ernest Augustus

CHAPTER 1

Craig's Story (The Why)
Take care of you for them.

Monday morning brekkies are always my favourite way to start the week. My buddies and I have been meeting for this "tune up" for almost a quarter of a century. We have so much fun and I'm sure that the other restaurant patrons just want to see us go home, coz the laughter can get pretty wild at times.

I often show pictures from my "Before and After" binder to people I start training. Mainly I do this for motivation and inspiration... but primarily to encourage nutritional and training adherence.

On one such day back in 1998, Craig started our morning conversation with, "I need to get in shape and I want to do the Body for Life Transformation Contest, and I want you to train me." We all burst out laughing. I could hardly catch my breath! Now you have to know that Craig is "the jokester" in our little group. Everything that comes out of his mouth is hilarious and no one takes him seriously.

So after I wiped the tears from my eyes I said, "Oh really? You're already in shape. Round IS a shape!" He actually looked at me with a straight face, not something I see often, and came back with, "Yeah, really!"

I thought I may as well play his silly little game so I said, "Ok, tell you what. How about right after brekky, you go over to the Dollar Store and pick up a little note pad. Then you write down EVERYTHING you put into your face for this upcoming week and bring the pad for next Monday's brekky for a little looksee, ees goot ya?"

I never in a bazillion years thought that he would do it. In fact, the following Monday, as we sat down at our favourite table, Craig threw a pad in front of me and I asked, "What's that?"

"That's what you asked me to do," he announced proudly.

"Oh right." I picked up the book and thumbed through it. I was pretty impressed but after a couple of minutes I asked him, "Would you like the good news or the bad news first?"

He looked at me and pleaded, "Geez man, prop me up. Give me the good news first!"

I congratulated him. "Craig, I'm super proud of you. I didn't think you would do it!"

He grinned from ear to ear. "Ok when do we get started?"

At which point I told him, "Whoa, don't forget the bad news. I'm looking at your first meal of the day last Monday and you had more fat in that meal than you're going to get for a whole week!"

"Lemme see, what'd I have?"

"You had two fried eggs, two pieces of toast with butter, deep fried hash browns and four strips of bacon. Not baby portions either, if I recall."

His only reply was, "You mean I have to give up bacon?"

"Oops, wrong word Craig! You don't HAVE to give up anything. You GET to give up bacon. Bacon is a heart attack on a plate!"

He looked dejected. "Ok I guess I can do that," he said.

I wasn't totally sold and told him so. "Let's do one more thing. For next week I need you to share with me a really good reason for you to do this. Your health and fitness isn't a game. This is going to be a huge step in your life journey, one that will take dedication and persistence. Craig, if you don't have a compelling reason, when that first road block appears in front of you - and believe me, it WILL show up and try to take you down - you won't be able to smash through it, get over it, or get around it. It'll stop you dead in your tracks. You'll look outside your window on a stormy winter day and say, 'Nah I don't want to scrape the car, I'll just skip the playground today'. You'll quit. That's not good enough, that's not the attitude that gets results."

The very next Monday Craig didn't even let me sit down at the table. "I put a lot of thought into it and I have my reason!" he said. "When my boys were young, we were very active. We used to play hoops, bat a ball around, kick a soccer ball, you know, lots of good active stuff. Well I have twin girls now and when they come to me and ask me to go for a bike ride with them, I can't get my fat butt off the couch! I'm tired of disappointing them, and myself. I want to do it for my girls."

"Craig," I said. "That's the most powerful 'why' I've heard in a long, long time!"

Now, poor Craig wasn't quite off the hook yet. When we got into the playground the following week he was experiencing a "snot-bubble blowing" barbell bench press "final burn out rep". From my spotter's position I yelled, "Craig, we need one more rep for Dara!" He actually squeaked out another wobbly rep, to which I ordered, "Oops, we just lost cabin pressure, but we still need one more rep for Kelly!"

Craig got amazing results!

Transferable Life Skill

Think about the REAL reason you're aiming for the goal. Sometimes the reason that you sabotage yourself is because you really aren't passionate about the goal. It's best to find a goal that you feel truly emotional about, to stay the course. I firmly believe that the passion of your "Why" is what eliminates procrastination and drives self-discipline and persistence to achieve the goal. If it don't really matter… it don't really matter! Have a good "Why"!

CHAPTER 2

Garry's Story (Priorities)

Take care of yourself so you have more to give

We were sitting in the office. I had just gone over his medical history and his exercise experience when he blurted out, "Actually I don't have a lot of time to exercise."

To which I replied, "Really, is that a fact? What fits your schedule better... exercise an hour a day, or being dysfunctional or dead twenty four hours a day?"

Ignoring me, he reached into his pocket and pulled out his business card. "I'm not trying to brag, but I'm a very busy guy and I have houses in Phoenix, Palm Desert and just over here close to the gym. I'm not even in town all the time."

I looked at his card. He was the developer of the largest high rise complex in the city. When I turned the card over, it showed five other high rises. "Garry, I've been training people since 1974 and I have to tell you that I'm always shocked by those people who will sacrifice their health to earn a ton of money, and once they have that money, they will pay anything to get their health back!"

He looked down sheepishly and said, "Yeah, that's really why I'm here."

"Ok, always remember that you're Priority Number One! If you don't have your health, you don't have anything. Who cares how much money you have if you can't enjoy it? Also, you're no good to anyone, your family, your business, no one, unless you're healthy and functional.

"When you're flying to one of your houses in Phoenix or Palm Desert, remember what they tell you on the plane if the cabin loses pressure. ALWAYS put your own oxygen mask on first! That's because you're useless to anyone else if you're incapacitated! Take care of yourself so you have more to give!"

I see Garry in the playground regularly. He's very consistent and his results show it. He's lost body fat and his energy levels are through the roof.

Transferable Life Skill

It can be very difficult to put yourself first. Especially for men, who all their lives have been told that they shouldn't be artists, or musicians, that they must sacrifice their dreams to support a family. They have no option but to work. If you have people that you are responsible for, YOU are the top priority. You MUST take care of you first or you're no good to your family, your company, or anyone! Allow me to rephrase an old motto for Ford Motor Company... "You're Job One!"

CHAPTER 3

Kalee's Story (Core Values)

Take responsibility for your health
now or be forced to later

Kalee was having a hard time making exercise a priority. "I'll find any excuse in the book to avoid it if I can. Sorry I'm late but at least I got here."

"Man, I'm going to kill you!" I teased as I pointed to my watch. "Three minutes late! Kalee, do you have any idea how much you've wrecked my day?"

"Sorry, I can't get up earlier to be here on time. It's so early," she said.

"You can't, or you won't, get up earlier?" I asked. "And what do you mean early? It's eight am. Eight hours of the morning have already gone by! How much sleep did you get last night?"

"I got my usual seven hours."

"So you went to bed around midnight? You don't have to answer this, but what the heck do you do until midnight?"

"I like to watch TV until I get sleepy."

"Kalee, TV is not your friend. It's a total time suck! Does it contribute to your personal life, your dreams, goals, aspirations, or is it just a bad habit? No one ever got to the end of the road and said, 'Gee, I wish I would have spent more time watching tv!'

"You should be cutting out all screen time at least an hour before going to bed, including cell phones and computers. The blue light emitted from the screens has been shown to disrupt the hormone melatonin which is your sleep hormone. It also suppresses delta brainwaves and boosts alpha brainwaves. Not a great idea for recovery, brain flushing, hormone balancing or just getting things done the next day."

"Yeah, you explained that to me once. What can I do?"

She opened the proverbial door, so I walked in. "I think you have your priorities screwed up. Perhaps you need to examine your core values to establish what's truly important."

"OK this sounds like another one of your life lessons. I think I have pretty good core values. I'm honest, opened minded, respectful..." she said.

"You're ABSolutely right. Those are some of your best features to be sure. But I'm going to put a spin on this for you. I might be wrong but I doubt it. If you were to be truly honest, open minded and respectful... of yourself, you would be respecting your health and your fitness a lot more, which would lead to other core values like commitment, reliability, determination and consistency, which in turn will lead to great results in everything you do."

Transferable Life Skill

It's very wise to analyze your core values - what you're truly made of, what you respect, and what you would like to be known for. Then align your goals with those principles that have the most meaning. Don't forget to factor in standards such as consideration for others or perhaps punctuality, that may not appear to be actual core values, but contribute to the overall picture.

CHAPTER 4

Jann's Story (Quality vs Quantity)

Live a life of no regrets

The playground in her condo building was being renovated so we started training in her condo unit. Jann is a "high performance" octogenarian. She had a stability ball, Power Blocks, a Bosu ball and various other goodies. A serious gal to be sure. She climbed Mt. Kilimanjaro when she was seventy five years old, bungee jumped off Victoria Falls in Africa the next year and went sky diving the following year! As I said – HIGH performance!

She notified me that there was only one reason that I was there. That was because her former trainer, of the last four years, was moving to Vangroovy and she needed someone else to terrorize her.

One day, a few months into our training, we had just finished a session in her unit and she excused herself to check the plumbing while I picked up the extra equipment that I had brought to the party.

After her bathroom break she said to me, "Come here!"

I was thinking, "Uh oh!"

She steered me into her bedroom and I was thinking, "Double uh oh!"

But then she pointed to pictures on her bedroom wall. "The reason that you're here is so that I don't have to go off this planet on that bed. I want to go out on one of those adventures." There were pictures of Jann on top of Mt. Kilimanjaro, white water rafting on the Burnside River, on horseback in Mongolia and other great life-time adventures.

Jann epitomizes my feeling that you never want to experience life from the outside looking in. You want to be right in the middle squeezing the freakin' juice out of it!

She's THE poster girl for living life to the fullest!

Transferable Life Skill

We were meant to move! Don't let anything hold you back. Live a life of adventure! Life is so short... make a difference. Make your contribution to this planet. Go for it! You never know when the sofa's going to land on your head!

CHAPTER 5

Tracy's Story (How Fit)

The weak get eaten

Because a number of my clients are lawyers, a few years ago I was doing "Health and Fitness" seminars for law firms. After a particular session was over and I was answering questions, Tracy asked, "How fit do you have to be?"

I assured her, "You don't have to be a fitness model or a body-builder. BUT... you should be fit enough to survive!"

Her "inner lawyer" escaped. "Explain!"

"Let's suppose this building was engulfed in fire. All the exits are blocked. We aren't going to smash the windows and jump fourteen floors down to the ground! That's not surviving. However, let's say some kind soul on the floor above us cuts a hole in the ceiling and lowers a rope. Are you fit enough to climb up that rope and save your sorry butt? If not, you're Kentucky fried... sorry... not fit enough to survive!"

She added, "Well, I guess I'm cooked."

I got it and followed up. "Ok, you may relate better to this. Let's say that you're going for a nice hike in the woods on a beautiful summer day with your best friend. Suddenly you come right between mama bear and baby bear. Not a good place to be! Mama bear rears up on her hind legs and charges toward the two of you! Can you out run your friend? If not, you're bear food... sorry... not fit enough to survive!"

"I'm still cooked," she admitted.

"I once read in a survival book that the aircrew is 'profiling' when you step onto their plane. They're looking for young fit men and making a mental note of where they sit. They can probably count on them to help in the event of an emergency. But they're also making a note of where the older obese people sit as well, because they will likely need the most help."

Transferable Life Skill

My dad told me to always do more than you're asked to do. It's easy to turn in a mediocre performance, phone it in so to speak, but at the end of the day, that may not serve you like you hope.

CHAPTER 6

Trisha's Story (Cost of Leanness)

Train like those who have what you want

Trisha and I were having a little chat in the cardio area while she was on her elliptical trainer. "How much work is it going to take to get in shape?" she asked.

My sales background kicked in. "Trisha, what kind of shape would you like to be in?"

She responded with stars in her eyes. "Well, of course, I want to look ripped!"

I thought I'd better read her the riot act. "Everybody would like to look like a fitness model; lean, toned, fit and radiant. But the real question is how many people are willing to pay the price?"

"I'm prepared to pay," she said.

"How much?" I asked. "The major law of the universe is the Law of Cause and Effect – 'What you put in is what you get out'. And therein lays the problem. People want to get something for nothing, or at least, for very little work.

"I'll tell you right now. It doesn't work that way. If you don't want much, you don't have to do much. If you want it all, you have to quit whining, put on the big-girl panties and suck it up. Just as with everything else in life, there's a cost. In this case, it's called the 'Cost of Leanness'. People will pay lip service and say that they'll do whatever it takes to be single digit body fat. But when it comes down to it, they don't want to do the work it takes, which can be considerable, which means they really don't want it bad enough."

"Ok, now you're scaring me," she said.

I continued. "Here's what I mean. If you want to be 'average', which at this time in human history is overweight at best, obese at worst. You don't have to do much. Keep shoveling truckloads of garbage into your face and lay on the sofa.

"However, let's say that you want to achieve 'a healthy body composition'. Now we're talking hitting the playground six times a week for an hour each session. You eat cleaner, getting more protein, fruits and veggies. You eliminate processed foods. You limit alcohol to once every week or two. You get seven to eight hours of sleep a night."

Thoughtfully, she put her hand on her chin. "Sounds do-able."

In my best infomercial voice I said, "But wait, there's more! Let's say you ABSolutely just have to have that fitness model's bod. Well here's what you get to do now. Prior to your photo shoot, you hit the playground twice a day for at least an hour each visit. You measure and weigh your food. You follow a macronutrient ratio protocol with more protein than a starving lion on the Serengeti can even look at. You carb cycle or at least carb taper. You cut out all fun foods. You cut salt. You eliminate alcohol. You choose social engagements carefully because you can only eat certain foods. And you have to go home early because you sleep at least eight, possibly nine hours a night to repair tissue."

"Yeah, I better weigh this one out," she said.

I looked at her. "Where do you draw the line? What are your priorities? Only you can answer these questions."

Transferable Life Skill

Decide how much you're prepared to sacrifice to get the results you want. Are you happy to just make ends meet, pay the bills and work a nine to five, or do you want to be a billionaire, jet setting and owning companies? Or perhaps well off is the aim. Be prepared to work extra hard for extraordinary results. Remember the First Law! What you put in is what you get out. Ask yourself what you're prepared to do, and what will never happen during your lifetime.

CHAPTER 7

Mandy's Story (Ease/Impact Grid)

The more you do – the more you get

"There's way too much to do to get healthy and fit. It's overwhelming. Where do I start?" Mandy asked.

I agreed. "You're so right, Mandy. Let me tell you that one of my all-time fave clients and personal friends, Tema Frank, has written a book... *People Shock*. In it she talks about the 'Ease/Impact Grid'. Now this is brilliant, so pay attention.

"Essentially she explains that there are some things that are easy to do that create little impact, and some that create huge impact. Then some things are hard to do that create little impact, and some create huge impact."

"This is so confusing. Thanks for that!" Mandy said.

"Sorry. Here's an example. If you really want to kick off your new weight loss program with a bang, do easy things that get great results."

"For instance?" she asked.

"Well, I wouldn't start measuring and weighing food yet. You get a huge impact from doing those things but it's not as easy as say, cutting starchy carbs for a noticeable result. Or you could start a walking program after dindin every night. Pretty easy to do, but considerably less impact than progressive training six days per week," I explained.

Ease/Impact

Easy – Small impact - Walking

Easy – Huge impact – Eliminate starches

Hard – Small impact – Eliminate salt

Hard – HUGE impact – Progressive training six days a week

Transferable Life Skill

Obviously a good way to start a job is to implement some easy projects first that will deliver huge impact. That'll get the ball rolling and create a feeling of movement. Take that movement and generate momentum which will help get you through the harder tasks. When it gets down to the fine details, you will have already created great results and only need to fine tune. Keep in mind that it can be grueling to nail down those fine details, but you're on a roll so it makes things really worth it.

CHAPTER 8

Frank's Story (SMART)

Accountability is the glue that ties commitment to results

"This transformation thing seems so unattainable. I have so much work to do and I just don't know where to start," Frank said as he stared at his rather substantial girth in the mirror.

"I think the first step might be to establish your goal," I suggested.

"Sure. I'd like to look like Arnold," he said half-jokingly.

"Howzbout we get SMART about this thing?" I asked.

"Are you saying I couldn't look like him?"

I explained, "You might. But I'm referring to the acronym SMART for goal setting. **S**pecific; you just can't say you want to look like Arnold. You have to define exactly the differences between you and him and the changes that you need to make. **M**easurable; it's got to be quantifiable. No guesses. You're going to be keeping really detailed records. **A**ttainable; you can't go after something like being 6'2" if you're 5'9". **R**ealistic; if you can't train six hours a day and eat chicken breasts until you grow feathers and peck gravel, it's not going to happen. And **T**imed; you have to set some short term and long term goals with deadlines.

"Goals are the gun. Deadlines are the trigger. Without them there's no sense of urgency and procrastination will rear its ugly head. Set a date to achieve the goal. Mark it in your calendar. Every time you see or hear that date it will trigger recognition neurons that will propel you forward."

A light bulb went off and Frank looked confident. "Great. Sounds like a plan!"

Transferable Life Skill

You need to have a plan for everything you do in life. Don't just wing it. With every goal… get SMART!

S - Specific

M – Measurable

A – Attainable

R – Realistic

T – Timed

CHAPTER 9

Deidre's Story (Dosage)

Don't wish it were easier – wish you were better

"I only want to train once every second week instead of once a week," she announced during our session.

"Can I ask what you're thinking?" I asked.

"I don't seem to be getting stronger," she responded.

A little shocked, I said, "Deidre, you do realize that we train with weights one Friday, then core the next Friday, and stretch the next Friday, at your request?"

"Yeah, I was hoping that would be enough," she replied.

"Here, please allow me this analogy. If your dentist was doing your semi-annual checkup and all of a sudden, mid stride, he stopped, and with a horrified look, shook his head and said, 'Houston, we have a problem here. How often do you brush your teeth?'

"And you said, 'I brush the tops one Friday, the bottoms the next Friday, and then I skip a Friday and start the routine over again.' I think that might explain why you aren't getting the results you want," I suggested.

She laughed. "Aw, c'mon, get real!"

I continued, "Using another example, if your doctor gave you a bottle of antibiotics for a nasty infection, but instead of following the directions of one a day, you decided to take only one pill a week for two weeks and then skip the third week, you would have taken two pills in the entire three weeks. That might be the very definition of 'ineffective dose'!

"People who want to transform their bodies can't get away with minimal training. In fact, their training is more like getting a jet plane into the sky. Full thrust is required to get off the ground until you reach cruising altitude, at which point you hit maintenance, where it gets easier to stay in the air and you can then pull back a bit. The toughest part is the beginning. And one third throttle will never get you off the ground. Can you say... 'sub optimal'?"

"So how often should I train?" she asked.

"You should be doing resistance training progressively three times a week in order to see the strength gains that you set as your goal when we first started. Not once every three weeks, never mind once every six weeks, as you're suggesting. Cardio another three times a week would be helpful as well," I advised.

She just looked at me and gulped!

Transferable Life Skill

You must have a consistent and regular plan with enough challenge to achieve adaptation and to actually make a difference. There is no "magic pill" that you can take to become successful, at anything. The only place where "success" comes before "sweat" is in the dictionary! Make no mistake! At the end of the road, TANSTAAFL (There Ain't No Such Thing As A Free Lunch!) Eventually you pay for everything. Your results will always be in direct proportion to your effort and that always entails the correct dosage.

CHAPTER 10

Rachel's Story (The Scale)

Focus on what has to be done

After assessing a member's exercise history, medical history and any deterrents, I always ask for a specific goal that we can work towards, something that is SMART (specific, measurable, achievable, relevant and timed). In most cases they will answer the question like Rachel.

"I'd like to be 110 pounds," she said.

Now that meant that she would have needed to lose 15 pounds. On a 5'7" female, her 125 pounds was just fine.

I looked at her and challenged her. "If you were exactly the same weight that you are now, but you dropped 3 dress sizes would you really care what your weight was?"

"Heck no," she answered quickly.

"Then weight is not the issue here is it? It's really body composition. How much fat you're carrying, right?"

Bewildered, she asked, "Yeah that sounds logical, but how's that going to happen?"

"The reason you can weigh more and look thinner is because a pound of fat is light fluffy material that takes up a lot of space whereas muscle, on the other hand, is compact dense material, and the same pound takes up less than 1/2 the space. You could have two people with identical bone structure, same height, same weight, and they could look entirely different. One looks fat and out of shape, the other looks fit and toned."

"Ok, let's lose some fat!" she cried.

"Now you're talkin'!"

Transferable Life Skill

The priority is not what it seems at times. When you really study the subject, you may find that you require a different way to look at the goal.

CHAPTER 11

Daphne's Story (Fear)

Fear and faith both require you believe in something you can't see

We were sitting in the office preparing to fire up a new program for Daphne. As I looked at the old program that I had made for her a couple of months before, I asked, "Daph, can you do pull ups now?"

"Well, you had me doing assisted pull ups, and every once in a while I would take the knee platform away and do a rep or so without the assist," she said proudly.

"FUNtabulous! UROCK!" I congratulated her. "Let's go out there and do some pull ups!"

"I'll go and get my bench," she said as she turned away and headed for the floor.

"Whoa, Daph. What do you need a bench for? This isn't a bench exercise. We're doing pull ups!" I said.

"So I can stand on it to grab the bar. I can't reach the bar."

"Ah, actually you can."

"No, it's too high."

"Ah, actually not. Come with me," I said as we headed for the pull up station. "Just put your hands up as high as you can under the bar and tell me how far you have to jump to reach it."

After half an attempt she said, "About three inches."

"Ok, so what's you're vertical?" I asked.

"My what?"

"You know... a basketball vertical jump. How high can you jump straight up? Now before you answer... you know that Michael Jordan can fly, right?" I was trying to encourage her will to win.

She hesitated. "I... I don't know."

"Then don't limit yourself. Just jump up and grab the bar."

"Ok, I'll try."

After two attempts she panted, "Not gonna happen."

I could see she had told herself that she couldn't do it, so I said, "Anyone can tell you I'm not great at math but I think you're a few feet short of Michael's flight path, yeah?"

After another failed attempt, I told her to jump as high as she could and touch the bar with one hand. "And look how nice I am to you. Your choice, whichever hand you like."

She did, and touched the bar with her right hand.

"Great! Now again. Jump up. Just touch the bar with the other hand."

She did.

"Super! Now touch it with both hands."

She did.

"Now grab the bar with both hands," I instructed.

A couple more tries and she got it. I told her to just hang on until she couldn't hang on any longer. "Dead hang. Get a mind-muscle connection. Feel your lats. Feel your biceps. Those are the muscles you need to recruit for this exercise."

After she dropped down to the ground, she looked at me and said, "Wow, I never thought I could do that!"

"You haven't seen anything yet!" I assured her as I passed her her water bottle. "Here, let me buy you a drink.

"Now jump up and grab that bar and dead hang. But this time, bend your knees and I'll cup my hands underneath them and assist you for a couple of reps... just like the assisted machine!"

Again, she did it. By the huge smile on her face I could tell that she was tickled with her accomplishment.

"Ok, while you're looking so happy... jump up. Grab that bar and show me your pull up!"

She started to knock them off, one by one. I started screaming in the playground. "Go Daph, go!"

Everyone stopped to watch. It was like a movie. The place went silent as everybody witnessed Daphne's history-in-the-making.

After three or four reps, and sticking the landing, she looked over to me grinning from ear to ear. Big Mike walked over, pointed straight at her and said, "THAT was awesome!"

Daphne looked at me proudly, her whole body vibrating. "Wow! That felt good!"

Val, who had been watching from the rail, walked over and said, "Daphne, I've always wanted to do pull ups and never thought I could. You just inspired me to try again."

I addressed them both. "Daph had a NOcebo. Exactly the opposite of a placebo (where your mind makes you believe something will work that really shouldn't). The NOcebo makes your mind not believe something will work that should work."

After our session she said, "That was really great! Thanks for the great work out and the super lesson!"

"Daph, it was a lot better for me than you could ever imagine. Just to see you beat your negative programming made my day. I thank YOU! Always remember: Your greatest fear is you! Fear is a choice!"

Transferable Life Skill

It has been said that when it comes to worry... 40% of all worries are never going to happen, 30% are over and in the past, 12% are needless worries about our health, 10% are petty miscellaneous worries, and only 8% of worries are legitimate and can be dealt with.

NEVER limit yourself. You are capable of way more than you think. And therein lays the crux. If you think you can and you try your hardest, it's amazing how many times you can do it. But if you think you can't and you won't even try, that's when you fail. The only time you fail is when you quit trying.

Visualize! See yourself succeeding! If someone else can do it, you can do it. You just have to figure out how. Then train and do it!

Theodore Roosevelt once said - "Far better it is to dare mighty things, to win glorious triumphs, even though checkered by failure than to take rank with those poor spirits who neither enjoy much nor suffer much, because they live in the gray twilight that knows neither victory nor defeat".

CHAPTER 12

Zoe's Story (Mental Blocks)

We're designed to win but some people program themselves to lose

Zoe was brand new to the playground scene. She was a 28 year old mom who had been a runner and played some recreational sports with her friends, but had never stepped in to a gym.

I was coaching her through a seated leg press for her program when she looked at me in sheer horror as I pinned half her body weight on the stack. "What are you doing? Are you trying to kill me?" she said.

"Not today... maybe next time. What's the prob?" I asked.

She stuttered, "Well...th... that's a lot of weight... isn't it?"

"Zoe... did you have brekky this morning?"

"Yeah."

"And did that occur at your kitchen table?"

"Yeah."

"And are you still sitting there?"

"Obviously not."

"Well to get up from the kitchen table, you had to fire exactly the same muscles to get your full weight out of the kitchen chair. They're huge muscles, the biggest in your entire body. This is only half your body weight. It should be a nice little warm up."

"Oh, yeah. Ok, that makes sense," she said as she broke through the mental block and easily pressed the platform through her full range of motion.

She also broke through the same mental block when she warmed up with half her weight on her calf lift as I explained, "You can easily stand on your tip toes, which is your entire body weight while peeking over the fence at your neighbors arguing in their back yard, right?"

Transferable Life Skill

As with Nocebos (see Chapter 11 – Daphne's Story) mental blocks can slow your progress in all areas of your life. Don't let that which doesn't make good sense hold you back in anything.

CHAPTER 13

Trudy's Story (Reframing)

Your greatest power is the power to choose

Trudy had just completed her fifth set of a six set progressive routine of seated tricep extensions. Her excruciating poop face indicated that she was entering the "level-nine" intensity territory. "Wow! That was really hard. Do I have to increase the weight on the next set?"

To which I replied, "Trudy, you don't have to do anything! You *get* to increase the weight for your final set! There are folks in the playground right here, who would LOVE to be able to increase the weight on *any* set! Take Tina over there. She's got MS. She would kill to be able to do your program. Every rep is a gift! You can thank me later!"

I'm not sure that she was totally convinced or wanted any gifts, especially from me. So I followed up. "Trudy, please tell me that's not the way you got through med school! When things got tough, you just gave up?"

She didn't answer and grabbed the heavier weight!

A great poster in my playground says, "Don't quit when you're tired... quit when you're done!"

Transferable Life Skill

Sometimes you need to change your perspective and reframe. If you ever catch yourself feeling sorry for yourself and you don't want to do something that you know you should, consider those who would love to but can't. And always maintain an attitude of gratitude!

CHAPTER 14

Ken's Story (Possibility Thinking)

You'll see it when you believe it

I have a friend who, as Zig Zigglar would say, "Has stinkin thinkin and needs a checkup from the neck up."

One night we were driving out of the parking lot that he "knew" very well. "You're never going to be able to turn left onto the avenue from here!" he warned.

Ignoring him, I approached the driveway. I looked both ways and drove immediately onto the road. No problem.

The next time, we're driving to the playground and I say, "Oh geez, I forgot to pick up something. Let's stop at Wally's World."

He shrieks. "Wally's World won't be open at this time!"

Again, ignoring him, I pulled into the parking lot. I walked right in to buy my stuff. No problem.

Then one night we're downtown and I said, "Hey, let's stop in and grab dindin at the Diner!"

"It'll be way too busy. Hansel will never want to see us at this time of night," he warned.

I parked the car right in front of the restaurant, went through the doors and Hansel came up to us and greeted us warmly. The place was a quarter full. No problem.

"In everything we do, possibility thinking is your friend! NEVER limit yourself!" I suggested.

"I didn't realize that I thought like that," he said.

"Most people don't. They're not 'possibility thinkers'. You have to look at EVERYTHING you do through the filter of possibility. Your question should always be – how can I? Not – 'I can't do that'. Don't limit yourself. I believe it was Henry Ford who said, 'Whether you think you can or you think you can't – you're right'"

Transferable Life Skill

The word "C-A-N-'-T" is NOT in our vocabulary! There may be times when something is difficult at the moment, but with analysis, perseverance, determination and commitment you can get the job done! Remember - believe you can and you're half way there! This is the reason why great people do great things, things that others told them was impossible. Then as Nike says, "Just DO it!" You'll be amazed at what you're really capable of doing when you adjust your thinking! This is so true in the playground, and in life.

CHAPTER 15

Doc Franklin's Story (Recording)

Consistent acts of excellence is the secret

Doc Franklin was doing his very best "Charlie Brown" imitation. You know the one. He's sprawled out on the floor with arms and legs spread out as if being drawn and quartered right after Lucy pulled the football away, just as he was about to kick it. "Gee, every session is hard," he groaned. "Does it ever get easier?"

I kneeled down on the floor beside him and whispered in his ear. "Nope, and you wouldn't want it to either!"

His sigh was so loud everyone in the playground looked around to see if he had expired.

"Now, let me show you your progress," I said as he sat up. He looked at his chart and saw that he had started that particular program two months ago. During that time he had increased his lifting capacity by a minimum of 70 percent in all muscle groups, and over 100 percent in his large muscles.

"I'm really glad you keep good records," he said, almost thankfully. "The program feels just as hard to do every time we get together."

I nodded. "And it is! That would be due to our progressions. If we were to go back to the very first time you did this program and use those weights that you said were a level nine intensity, you would pick them up today and laugh your way through all the sets. It's called adaptation and conditioning."

I then offered him a goodie. "Geoff, we still have five minutes left in our session. Would you like to knock off some Killer Abs with me?"

To which he replied, "Randy, I'm hot. I'm tired. And I'm sweaty. I just want to go home!"

Transferable Life Skill

Keeping really good records starting from the beginning will not only tell you how far you've progressed, but it will also tell you what's working and what's not working. Recording your training progress and your nutrition intake is an extremely valuable tool. Use this tool in your business and your projects to always know where you are, where you're going and how far you have left to go to acquire the goal. As Peter Drucker, the business guru said, "You can't manage what you don't measure."

CHAPTER 16

Jada's Story (Precision)
Don't just change - progress

"How accurate is this measurement?" Jada asked as we completed her body composition analysis.

I explained. "There's only one 100% accurate method to determine body fat. We don't use this method because it's extremely painful. It's called an autopsy!

"Now there are other methods as well but again, they're not 100% accurate either.

She looked confused. "Like what?"

"There's hydro static immersion. More affectionately known as the 'dunk tank'. You sit in a sling scale, expel your breath and the clinician drops you into a big vat of soup. Through mathematical equations using Archimedes' principle, they calculate your body fat. You can usually get this done at the university for a fee. But it's not 100% accurate because most people hate drowning so they retain a bit of air in their lungs and skew the readings.

"What else?" she asked.

"Well there's DEXA, Dual Energy Xray Absorptiometry. But it's not 100% accurate because it's mainly designed to measure minerals and lean soft tissue. It indirectly calculates fat mass, so it can provide some skewed results.

"Or you could stand on a bioelectric impedance scale and let it shoot a little electric current through you (not enough to make your hair stand on end). The machine computes the time it takes to receive the signal and through the built-in algorithms it determines your body fat. But the accuracy is dependent on hydration. If you're dehydrated or just had a case of beer, or maybe had a nice run around the block, the numbers will be off. So it's not totally accurate either.

"Now, here's the least invasive, least expensive, fairly accurate way to test your body fat. I pinch you with my pliers. It's a caliper test where I input the total millimeters of fat calculation into an equation after pinching you in a few body sites. In your case it would be the back of the arm, the shoulder blade, the love handle, the tummy and the thigh.

"But this method is subject to human error as well. I have to pinch you in EXACTLY the same spots three times every time we do the analysis. Unless we use a magic marker, that's hard to do.

"So really, there's nothing that we can do here that is 100% accurate. What you're looking for is a trend."

Transferable Life Skill

Unless you're a surgeon, a lawyer, or an engineer, don't fixate so much on details that don't make a difference. Look for trends.

CHAPTER 17

Debbie's Story (Goodwill Deal)

Do it with conviction

I always encourage my people to train for maximum health and functionality. Along with these come fitness and a healthy body composition. But there are other "benefits".

"Wow! I'm so happy. I've lost ten percent of my body fat and I'm gonna need a new wardrobe soon!" Debbie proudly declared.

"Pamfastic job Deb. Now here's the deal that I make with everybody. Now that your clothes are fitting too loosely, you HAVE TO take them to the Salvation Army or to Goodwill! Donate them! You're NEVER going to need them again. You'll NEVER cross that bridge again because you'll be in maintenance! DO NOT enable yourself to go backwards!" I told her. "If you know you have 'fat clothes' hiding in the closet, it can be a slippery slope right down to the bottom of the hill."

"But I paid a lot of money for some of those suits!" she whimpered.

"Do you have a tailor?" I asked. "You can have the expensive clothes taken in, and the excess material cut off so they can never be let out again! Deal?"

"Deal!" she replied.

A new wardrobe can be a huge motivator and a real bonus for some folks!

Transferable Life Skill

Never allow yourself the option of regressing. Eliminate all possibility of future failure. Burn the bridge!

CHAPTER 18

Jillian's Story (Variety)

Consistency turns average into excellence

Jillian had been referred to me by a friend. Her past trainer had been with her for a total of three years but had just moved out of town. I was sitting with her in the middle of our initial interview. "What type of programs did your other trainer prepare for you?" I asked.

She shrugged. "Well, we did something different every time we got together... there weren't really any two programs alike."

I shook my head. "Uh oh, this is going to be a deal breaker, Jillian. Can I assume that she was a lot younger than me?"

"Oh yeah, she's probably half your age, maybe a quarter," she laughed.

"Ok, please understand that I would never ever show any disrespect to your past trainer but there's a certain, what I call, 'Sesame Street mentality' that goes with some age groups. They were brought up watching things flashing at them very quickly on TV and they grew accustomed to that speed. Now, they tend to become bored with things quite easily. Then when some of these people become trainers, they have a tendency to change exercises and programs quickly, not because the client gets bored, but because they do."

"Ok, I get it."

"Now as you can see, I'm an old guy. I follow the Principles of Training. The first of which is the 'Adaptation Principle'. We'll continue to do the same exercises with progressions so that you acquire an adaptation response until we can't go further and incur the Ceiling Principle. This will also help prevent injuries!"

"I don't get it," she admitted.

"Well, think of it this way. If you were taking piano lessons and only played a particular piece once, how good would you get at it?" I asked.

"Not very," she said.

"Right. By starting with the initial part and layering more and more parts, then repeating the entire score a number of times, you acquire proficiency and your mind and body learns and adapts to the piece. Only then should you go on to a new, more intricate composition.

"So that's the way I work. We'll start with an exercise movement and slowly progress it until you achieve muscular and neural adaptation. Then once you're stronger and totally competent with that program we can ramp it up and challenge you even further with a new program."

"But don't you ever get bored?" she asked.

"I haven't been bored for... oh... prolly fifty years or so!" I responded honestly.

She nodded. "Ok, makes sense. Sounds good to me."

And that's when we started a most pamfastic training relationship.

Transferable Life Skill

When I used to play in bands I was always very disappointed in the band members who wanted to replace certain tunes in the set list just because they were bored of playing them. I had to remind them that we could play whatever we wanted when we rehearsed but that our fans and audiences wanted to hear the tunes we played that they had come to love. And they expected us to play them with the passion that they had paid for. We weren't playing for us... we were playing for them.

Change for the sake of change is not usually a great idea. Only after you've learned the necessary lessons is it wise to move on to a more challenging endeavor. If you're still learning and have more to learn, discipline and creativity can go a long way to achieving true success.

CHAPTER 19

Jan's Story (Open Mind)
The unknown is where adventure and possibility lives

One summer day we were visiting some friends at their lake cottage. Knowing that I terrorize people in the playground for a living, they were eager to show me their new "exercise equipment acquisition."

We walked into a room and there in front of us stood a full size vibration trainer. I hadn't seen a "vibration contraption" since the 1970s! I must admit, my crappo meter was the only thing "vibrating"!

"I use this every morning right after my rebounder. It keeps me in great shape. Wanna try it?" Ken said.

"I'm game. Let's give it a go!" I said. After a few minutes of rockin' and rollin', shakin' and shukkin', still very skeptical, I told him as humanely as possible, "It's a nice machine."

That was 2010. Fast forward to 2017 at the YMCA.

"Where are your vibration trainers?" Jan asked looking around the playground.

"We don't have any," I said. "I'm not sure they're very effective."

"You should research them," was all she said and walked away.

Later that week I was in the middle of my daily reading of one of the health and fitness web sites that I subscribe to and this particular article said that Mark Wahlberg's personal trainer takes a portable vibration trainer over to his house to train him. Apparently, according to the article, Dwayne "The Rock" Johnson uses one as well.

I was starting to think, 'Really? Is it possible? Or is this just some advertising gimmick?'

I thought to myself, 'Perhaps if a person actually DID their exercises on the vibration trainer, instead of just standing on the thing, hoping the fat was going to just shake away, it could create enough instability that it would fire stabilizers in a different way, and that was the reason that some movie stars would use it, and possibly get some results?'

But why not just use a stability ball or a Bosu ball?

Is it possible that the instability created by a Bosu or stability ball is 'predictable', so to speak? So as you create the instability, your body knows what it has to do to stabilize itself and starts to react in advance. The movement of a vibration trainer could be a 'surprise' to the body and cause a quicker firing of the muscles, similar to a reaction ball, as long as the trainer controls the movement.

So then I figured I'd go online and research vibration trainers. For it to have a hope of working there were three criteria that had to be met:

-It had to be big enough to hold a larger client

-It had to move in multiple directions, not just one, and

-It had to have a remote so that I control the 'surprise' to the client

Well, I bought one and then developed a very unconventional exercise program for it, incorporating stability balls and Bosus. I may write another book letting you know the results after the test drive.

Transferable Life Skill

Always keep your eyes open to different ways of getting the job done. Never say 'no' until you've actually given it the ol' college try to determine if it really works. Test drive everything! The science is NOT always in!

CHAPTER 20

Monica's Story (Hard-Easy)

Nothing great comes without effort

She looked up at me from her bench, steam pouring out of her ears, blood squirting from her eyes and a whole tub of snot bubbles erupting from her face. I think she got a level ten intensity.

"That was really hard!" she gasped.

"And you wouldn't want it to be easy either!" I smiled and congratulated her. "FUNtabulous job, Monica. If it was easy everyone would be doing it and everyone would look like a fitness model!

"The only way you can make your brain better is to challenge it. The only way to make your body better is to challenge it! You can't come into the playground and do a cakewalk.

"Little pink fuzzy weights are NOT your friends. Pick up some real iron! A walk in the park is NOT going to take you to your goal! You rock!"

Transferable Life Skill

The road to the top is not usually the smoothest. Very often there will be potholes and lots of ups and downs. But when you make it, the view is spectacular and definitely worth it!

CHAPTER 21

Bryan's Story (All or Nothing)

The real workout starts when you want to stop

"My problem is that once I start on a bag of chips I have to finish the whole bag. And then since I already blew my plan, I may as well just keep on eating. I sabotage myself," Bryan confessed.

"You're an 'all or nothing' person! That would be fat loss suicide!" I said.

"You know it. And it's so discouraging and difficult to start over and over again!" he said.

I was on a roll. "Try this. ONLY do one or two simple things at a time. People try to do too many things and they get overwhelmed. When they can't do it all, they feel like they failed and can never win. So they quit. But if you give yourself a break and only make one or two changes, it's a lot easier and the chances of completion are much greater.

"Here are a few simple changes. Pick one or two areas ONLY, to focus on:
- add more veggies to each meal
- add more water to your daily intake
- add more protein to your meals
- no skipping meals
- cut snacking after dinner
- wake up 10 minutes earlier
- eliminate one processed food
- eliminate one dessert a week

- run around the block one day a week

"Bryan, if you were taking the bus to Calgary and the wheels fell off. You wouldn't just turn around and walk home would you?" I asked. "No, you might sit by the side of the road and try to figure out what happened but then you'd put the wheels back on the bus and keep rolling! That's the trick to achieving any goal!

"Always try to remember your reason for wanting to reach the goal in the first place! You have to have a compelling reason!" I said.

He agreed. "I think I got it!"bh

Transferable Life Skill

All or nothing thinking can lead to the death strike! There will be constant "ups and downs" on the journey. It isn't a constant linear progression. Remember your "Why"! Why did you start it in the first place? Now DO something! And don't quit!

CHAPTER 22

Jamie's Story (Master Mind Group)

Be a gymaholic

"This is so hard to do by myself," Jamie said. "I'm not dissing you. I enjoy your company and all, but it would sure be nice to have a work-out bud."

I agreed. "I hear ya. Having a training partner can deliver twice the results. You don't want to let your partner down. So even if you're dragging your butt that morning you're going to show up at the playground. It works both ways and more consistent attendance is the outcome.

"Also, very often, there's that little bit of competition. Not with each other because there shouldn't be. But if your partner gets a personal best that morning it can be a huge motivation and inspire you to do the same."

"But, I don't know anyone who exercises besides me," she said.

"Tell ya what, Jamie. Point out a few people to me here in the playground who seem to be here when you are and I'll introduce you to them right now."

Transferable Life Skill

In Napoleon Hill's book *Think and Grow Rich*, he has an entire chapter devoted to "The Master Mind Group", in which he explains that "not one person can do or think of everything by themselves". Forming a group of people who have the same goals can utilize the talents of each individual to acquire results that move the entire group in the direction of their goals much quicker than the individual could on their own.

CHAPTER 23

Anna's Story (Time)

Excuses are for those who need them

"When is the best time to work out?" Anna asked, repeating a question that I hear often. "I don't have much time."

Oops. Now she got me started.

"Anna, you have all the time there is! Everyone has the same amount of time, twenty four hours in the day. It's what a person does with that time that determines their success in anything! If a person works eight hours and sleeps eight hours, that leaves eight hours a day to do other things. Now if we're talking priorities. Your health and fitness should be priority ONE because nothing else means anything without your health!"

"But I have a family to take care of," she said.

"How good are you to anyone if you aren't healthy? Do you think your family can get along well if you're sick?" I fired back.

"Well, I guess not."

"Now having said that, let me answer your first question. The best time of day to train is first thing in the morning for the following reasons:

Most people go to sleep at different times every night depending on what's happening in their lives, but they usually get up at the same time every morning. So getting up earlier is way easier to start a great repeatable habit.

Start the day off right. Get your circulation pumped. Raise your metabolism and grab a load of endorphins. A client, Trent, used to tell me that when he trained early in the morning with me, he could handle anything that came his way during the day. He was fired up.

But if he didn't train until later or not at all, it was way tougher to deal with everything that came his way, and energy was an issue for the whole day.

And here's the big one: it's very easy to skip a workout session after work because people are too tired, or they have a meeting, or they forgot about a family commitment or all kinds of other issues. So consistency can be really poor."

"But you get up at an ungodly hour to train don't you?" she asked.

"I've trained at five am six days a week for over forty five years," I said. "I look at it this way... five hours of the morning has already gone by. It's time to get up and start the day off right!"

Transferable Life Skill

Consistency is everything. Everybody has an excuse! Excuses don't get results! Excuses will kill you! Keep the goal in mind. Visualize and really feel yourself achieving the results that you initially wanted at the beginning of the journey. Set up a new more efficient routine.

CHAPTER 24

Marlene's Story (Doin' it Right)

The only thing standing in your way is you

One of my other volunteer positions was on the Communications Committee for my favourite charity, The Rainbow Society of Alberta. It grants wishes for children with life threatening conditions and severe chronic medical illnesses.

I had offered free training to a fellow who had entered the Body for Life Contest and had promised to donate any winnings to our kids. I figured the least I could do was help him win. Unfortunately, he had already completed ten of the twelve weeks so my two week involvement didn't help all that much.

At any rate, one day a couple of staff members and I were sitting in the office talking about the contest when Marlene, another volunteer, walked in and joined the conversation.

"The Body for Life Program didn't work for me. I tried it," she announced, as a matter of fact.

"How often did you switch up the program?" I asked, knowing that one of the problems that most people have is doing the same exercises for the entire twelve weeks.

"I… I went four weeks doing the same exercises and then I quit," she said, with a slight question in her voice.

"Oops, that was precisely when you were supposed to reverse the exercises in the program. What levels of intensity did you achieve?" I asked, again knowing that very few people ever reach the required intensity.

"What do you mean, levels of intensity?"

"Well, the program required that you train to a 'high point', a level ten intensity that would get those coveted micro tears in the tissue so that you could repair and gain muscle. What progressions did you use?" I asked.

"What do you mean progressions?" she asked, starting to realize that her attempt at the program was definitely sub optimal.

"If you're a newbie to exercise, more than likely, every time you train for the first few weeks, you can get 'personal bests' every time out. In other words, each time you stepped into the playground, you would have been able to increase the weights in each exercise slightly. Highly trained gym warriors aren't able to do that, although they would love to. I always push my newbies through admirable progressions the first few weeks. They're definitely very proud of their accomplishments in such a short time.

"How many 'cheat days' did you take on your nutrition plan?" I just had to hear the answer to this one.

"Uh, well," she hesitated.

I added. "People get it wrong most of the time. Either they skip 'cheat days' altogether, thinking that they will get faster results if they don't 'cheat' at all, or they end up taking too many 'cheat days'."

"Well I figured that instead of taking a 'cheat day' once a week, I would spread my six meals out and have a 'cheat meal' once a day. Oops."

Now she was starting to get the idea.

"I think, depending on the portion of your 'cheat meals', that you probably sabotaged your entire week of clean eating," I said. I was hoping that she might try again, but perhaps correctly the next time.

Transferable Life Skill

Make sure that you're on the right track. Study the procedure inside and out and stay the course. Get help if you need it, but don't quit if you know others have achieved their goals using the same method. It invariably works if you do it correctly.

CHAPTER 25

Ronnie's Story (Stay the Course)

If it ain't broke don't fix it – if it *is* broke – fix it

Ronnie was a little discouraged. "My goal was to lose more than 10 pounds this month, and I only lost eight."

"Ronnie, I only have this to say about that. One - you lost two pounds a week. The medical profession considers that to be ideal and sustainable. Congratulations! Two - we haven't done your body comp analysis yet. How do you know that you didn't lose more fat and put on muscle?"

She was almost crying. "But maybe I should try a different nutrition plan or change up my training."

"Whoa! Whoa! Not so quick. Let's do your body comp first to determine what you lost... and perhaps... what you've gained."

After pinching her with my pliers we discovered that she had, in fact, lost eight and half pounds of fat and put on a half-pound of muscle. A most commendable job.

She was still not satisfied (she's definitely a Type A personality).

"Should we change the program?"

"Based on what we both saw, my suggestion is that we stay with what worked. You definitely have the right idea Ronnie. If it's not working we have to change something, but think of it this way. If you continued to get these results, you would be down over 40 pounds of fat and have gained over three more pounds of muscle by year end. That's way ahead of your original goal."

"Can't we do it faster?" she blurted.

"Fersure, you want to lose a bunch of weight right this minute? I can remove your arm... or a leg... your choice," I joked.

"Listen, this whole journey is an experiment to find out what works for Ronnie. Everyone has different body chemistry, different metabolism, different gut biome, different muscle compositions, different absorption rates, heck, even the lengths of our levers are different. What works for one person doesn't necessarily work for another and vice versa. If we could find something that worked for everyone and bottle it, we would be bazillionaires. We've found something that works for you, although maybe not as quickly as you would like. Please, you're trying to have a poop before it's there!"

"Ok, I guess you're right. I didn't look at it that way. I'll hang in."

Transferable Life Skill

In the game of life... patience can be a virtue. Once you find something that works don't be quick to change it. Let it run its course until you achieve the goal or until it no longer works. Then change the goal or find another option. If the horse is still moving, stay on it!

CHAPTER 26

Joey's Story (Success Manual)

Believe in yourself

"Joey's eyes were filled with tears. "I'm just so down. I can't pull myself up and get myself to the gym. I feel like I'm failing at everything."

"Mom said there would be days like this," I said sympathetically. "Joey, have you ever heard of a 'success manual'?"

"No, what is it?" she asked through tiny sniffles.

"Well one of the major 'Laws of the Universe' is the Law of Rhythm - nothing is always up and nothing is always down. There's a flow to it. Up AND down. Even superstars have the occasional 'slump'. It's the law. The difference is, they know how good they truly are. So they only hit the low point for a very short time and then they get out of the funk and ride the high wave for a really long time.

"I used to be a volunteer co-facilitator for The City of Edmonton Community Services Men's Groups. One of the ways I would teach our guys to get out of a rut was to make a 'success manual'. My own is a nice leather binder, filled with all kinds of things I'm really proud of, thank you notes, certificates, pictures, cards, accomplishments, and things that remind me of what I'm truly capable of achieving.

"Joey, you need to make one for yourself. I'm sure that you can think of a lot of things right now that you're very proud of, things that really show your personal power."

"Like what?" she sobbed. "I can't think of anything right now."

"Well you started and run your own small business right? How many people have the guts to do that? You have a business degree.

That's a testament to your ability to stay focused and to go the distance. I've met your kids. They're super polite, accomplished, outgoing and well-balanced. You should be very proud.

"On your way home, promise me that you'll stop and pick up a binder so that you can start your success manual. But before you do, let's get out to the playground and fire up some endorphins to help the process!"

She perked up. "I promise!"

Transferable Life Skill

You will never truly appreciate the heights of the mountains until you have experienced the depths of the valleys. Understand the laws of the Universe. Make a success manual and when you get down on yourself, sit in your favorite easy chair, turn on some soothing music and go through it page by page. Relive everything and all the feelings you experienced. Know who you truly are. You're incredible! YouTube "Desiderata"!

CHAPTER 27

Yolanda's Story (Imagination)

This is the only body you're gonna get this lifetime

"Why can't I get into this?" Yolanda started to explain. "I've tried for years to really force myself. I mean, I just know that I'm not as keen on exercise as I should be, or as dedicated as you are."

I could see she was feeling dejected. "Well, we didn't have the same past lives," I joked. "I was very ill in one of my past lives and confined to a life of immobility in another. In this life I really appreciate my good health and my ability to function optimally. I don't ever want to lose either."

"C'mon, get serious," she pressed. "What about now? What really motivates you now?"

I decided to share my latest discovery with her. "When I had eye surgery, I was forced to quit my maintenance exercise routine for three weeks. It was the first time in over forty three years up to that time.

"I just knew it would be tough. So when the surgeon told me that she didn't want me creating excess pressure on my eye and I wasn't to lift more than 30 pounds during the recovery time, I informed her that it would be depressing at best, suicidal at worst."

Then I tried to bargain with her. "Does that mean 30 pounds all together? Or can that be 30 pounds in each hand?"

Eye roll! Her lack of humour was palpable. She was certainly not amused.

My nature doesn't allow giving up after the first attempt so I tried again. "Can I continue my training if I do these three things to relieve eye pressure? I promise to practice core bracing, proper breathing technique and time under tension. That should relieve pressure, right?"

She stared at me like I just grew another head right in front of her. "If you re-open that incision and it gets infected you could lose your eye!"

"Roger that! It was the longest three weeks of my life! After the type of training that I do, hour long walks just don't cut it! It felt like I was 98 years old! I could hear the muscle wasting away every minute of every day!

"However, during that time... during one of those stupid walks, actually, I came to the realization that the real reason I exercise six days a week is not to look strong and lean (the fact that I carry low body fat is merely a 'side benefit'). The real reason is because I just don't ever want to have heart disease or need a walker. Both of those scare the bejeebers out of me.

"Now, I know that you can't ever stop the dealer from dealing the cards and that the house will eventually win. But I say... stay in the game as long as you can and play the hand you're dealt as brilliantly as possible. Exercise, eat right and stay away from as many toxins as you can."

Transferable Life Skill

Sometimes imagining a life without something you should really be grateful for can help you to appreciate what you have. It should drive you to make sure that you never take it for granted and do everything in your power to hang on to it.

CHAPTER 28

Leia's Story (The Reason)

It's always a choice

"I'm really surprised that I'm here," Leia said, tongue in cheek.

"Where would you rather be?" I asked.

She assured me it wasn't me. "It's just that exercise is something I just don't think of doing, you know, for fun. I could be with my friends having laughs and a good time," she sighed.

"Yep, I suppose you could. But answer me this. How many laughs can you have and how much fun would it be if you were unhealthy, say in a hospital... or in a wheelchair?" I asked.

She shot back, "C'mon, you make it sound like if I don't exercise, the worst is going to happen to me."

"Well, the universe has weird ways of getting you to listen sometimes. A few weeks ago I was doing my CPR Recert and during the 'choking' part of the training, my partner let go of me and I ended up on my back. It was cranky for days. During my next workout I felt a pop during a dumbbell squat. I dropped the weights and dropped to my knees. The pain was excruciating. I could barely get up. But as I struggled to my feet, I thought, 'Yikes, what's the universe trying to tell me here? I better take really good care of myself if I want to continue in my profession, and... do I really want to cut out one buffet a week?'"

Transferable Life Skill

Things happen for a reason. Sometimes life takes a whole new path if you neglect the priorities. Hopefully, the path will lead to where you want to go. But it would be very wise to make sure you're on the right path in the first place.

CHAPTER 29

Jay's Story (What's that Smell?)

Fitness is not for the weak

Doc Jay looked up at me from his Bosu dumbbell Arnie Press, took a deep breath and said, "I stink!"

Now, you have to know that the good doc is pretty easy going. I was hoping he wasn't feeling too self-conscious, so I laughed and said, "If you aren't sweating in the playground, you're not having any fun! It's called 'Eau de Gym'... good things come to those who sweat!

"When a survey was done asking people where fat went when they exercised, very few knew the answer," I said.

"So where does it go?" he asked.

"It forms carbon dioxide and H_2O ie. sweat. So... you rock! Sweat is fat crying!"

Transferable Life Skill

Don't worry about the people around you who are phoning in their performance. Give it everything you've got and do it right. Better judged by twelve than carried by six. Another way to say this is... if you're not living on the edge... you're taking up way too much space.

CHAPTER 30

Kristie's Story (The Line)

Recalibrate

"I was doing great with my nutrition plan until Barry and I went to that darn concert," Kristi confessed.

"What happened there?" I asked.

"Barry takes off to go to the washroom... or so I thought. But he comes back with two giant hot dogs!" she said.

I looked at her quizzically. "So... you didn't have to eat the hot dog, right? You could have told him that either he could eat it or you could take it home in a puppy sack."

"I guess," she waffled.

"Look Kristie, you gotta draw a line in the sand somewhere. It's the line you just won't cross. It could be a body composition number or a number on the scale. As soon as you see that number, everything gets dialed up. Big time. And you go into 'damage control'."

She shot back, "But I DO have a number that I don't want to cross."

"I know. We've been working on keeping you behind that line for the last few months. Perhaps the line needs to be moved closer to allow for the odd lapse!"

Transferable Life Skill

You must have a point of no return. A place you can't go... morally, ethically, or with your health and fitness goals. You know where it is. Give yourself some cushion but adjust the line when things aren't working.

CHAPTER 31

Raquel's Story (It's Criminal)

Easy choices – hard life. Hard choices – easy life

Raquel is a judge... and while explaining ideas or principles to clients or members, I always try to refer to something they can relate to in their lives or fields of work.

One day we were in the middle of a HIIT session. She was doing her 16th one-minute plank (out of twenty) between resistance sets. She likes me to talk to her while she's in plank position, so I threw an idea at her that I'd been thinking about.

"I think that getting lean for the average person is analogous to a career criminal staying clean."

"How so?" she asked.

I continued, "Once a career criminal is back on the street, it's really hard for them to stay clean. They can't enable themselves by having drugs or weapons anywhere near them. They need to select their environment very carefully... and that means friends as well.

"A person whose goal is leanness can't enable themselves by having their cupboards full of twinkies or chocolate bars. And if they surround themselves with obese people whose idea of a good time is bar hopping and hitting Mickey D's at two in the morning... they're going right back to jail!"

She agreed. "That could be a little tricky. A person could relapse early on."

"Yep, but the goal is maintenance... where having the odd candy bar every so often is not going to kill all your efforts... just as seeing an old cell mate on visiting days is not going to turn you back into the life," I said.

Transferable Life Skill

This entire life journey is a matter of learning lessons. But it's not just the knowledge you acquire. You must understand how it all works together. Then you must apply the information. As Bruce Lee so wisely said, "Knowing is not enough, we must APPLY! Willing is not enough, we must DO!"

CHAPTER 32

Winnie's Story (Wrong Track)

Fail. Learn. Move through it. Repeat.

"Geez... this stupid thing!" Winnie said in frustration.

"What's happening?" I asked, watching intently as she struggled with her hoodie zipper after our playground session. Her zipper broke and after she "fixed" it and pulled it up... it meshed alright... but it wasn't "even" when she zipped it to the top.

We both had a good laugh as we looked at the final product.

"This is the story of my life," she said. "Including all the workout plans I've tried."

"I'm sure that you've tried a few but I wonder if you started them off the way you zipped your hoodie!"

"Like how? What do you mean?"

"You sorta missed the alignment on the zipper right at the onset," I said. "If you don't start any new program properly, the results will be less than optimal. It's the reason why so many people take their Ikea projects home and end up with extra pieces or something that looks nothing like the floor model or the picture on the box."

"It makes sense, but give me another example," she said.

"Ok, I know so many people who, through inattention to detail, or just plain laziness, have started a nutrition program without even learning what 'macro nutrients' are. They couldn't tell you the difference between a carb and a protein. But then they wonder why their 'clean eating' plan didn't work. Then they want to jump ship and try the newest thing that comes down the pipe."

Transferable Life Skill

Strategy dictates results. Winnie thought she started the zipper evenly at the bottom but she didn't, just like people who think they start a project correctly... but don't. They continue until they "pull the zipper to the top" and realize that it doesn't work.

Don't continue following the wrong path. Keep measuring to know when you're on or off target and adjust accordingly.

CHAPTER 33

Clara's Story (Details)

You can't lose by taking action

Clara would show me her exercise/nutrition log book every week when we got together, along with all kinds of health information she found on the internet. But she wasn't really very consistent with either the exercise or the healthy eating. And due to all the time wasted searching and not adhering to the program, she didn't get great results. After a few weeks I wondered when she was really going to come to the party and get on it.

"Clara, what exactly are you researching?" I asked.

"I've got to make sure that I'm doing all the best things. I don't want to do the wrong things," she answered.

I looked at her in amazement and asked, "Have you ever heard of that terrible disease, 'Analysis Paralysis'?"

"What do you mean?" she asked.

"I think you're rearranging the deck chairs on the Titanic," I suggested.

"Ok, now you're really confusing me," she admitted.

"Clara, you're majoring in minor things. While you rearrange the deck chairs, the ship is sinking. You're not getting optimal results because you stall out while you search for the silver bullet. Let me save you some time. There IS no silver bullet! Everyone is different. Different metabolism. Different body chemistry. Even the lengths of our levers are different, which could require a different personal exercise protocol. This is a journey, an experiment to find out what works for Clara. We gotta start someplace, but we gotta start."

Transferable Life Skill

There comes a time when taking action is paramount. Yes, research is wise, but only to the degree that it keeps you safe and starts you in the right direction. You can always change directions on route, but you have to start.

CHAPTER 34

Janaia's Story (Will Power)

Greatness is a habit

Being an old guy and very, very technologically challenged, I stay in touch with my family, friends, clients, and members through email.

One day I received this goodie from Janaia. "Hey coach, I was reading a book on 'habits' the other day and the author said that 'will power' is lower in the evening. I think this is definitely true for me and lots of other people. How can I overcome this?"

"Wow... there's the bazillion dollar question! I'm convinced that if everyone had super determination, discipline and self-control, our world would be a much better place. It would seriously cut into the 'Seven Deadly Sins'. That's for sure! Closer to home, trainers would be out looking for new careers because the two sins we address in our industry, 'gluttony and sloth' would have gone the way of the dinosaur," I told her.

She agreed.

I continued, "In answer to your question, I would start by first, eliminating the limiting belief that 'will power is lower in the evening'! If your conscious mind believes that's true, your subconscious mind will do a 'Captain Picard' on you, and 'make it so'.

"Second, I would be very conscious of when you crave, what you crave, and what emotions you're feeling when you do. Are you feeling bored, sad, angry, lonely, stressed, frustrated...? Become conscious of your subconscious. What is your emotional addiction? Are you getting a dopamine hit? Are you medicating with food?

"Then I would record all the information for further analysis. You might perhaps 'Google'... 'Why do I crave salty snacks late at night when I'm bored?' You'd be surprised at all the great advice you can get.

"You need to address the emotional issue and find a substitute for the indulgence," I added.

Transferable Life Skill

Understand that will power... self-discipline and self-control affects every area of your life. Ask yourself why you do, or don't do things that you know would help you achieve your goals.

Plato said, "The unexamined life is not worth living."

Earl Nightingale said that there are three things you must study: your business, your language, and people... that includes YOU.

In fact... YOU are the most important component. Focus your studies on YOU!

And while you're studying YOU, only study relevant positive information to make YOU the best YOU can be. No fluff or negativity. Do as all motivational speakers will tell you, stay away from newspapers. They sell sensationalism. No one needs to start their day with all that negative garbage! But if you're totally addicted to reading the newspaper, and you ABSolutely must wallow in your fetish, it's been said that if you want to see people doing their absolute worst, read the front page of the paper. If you want to see people trying their best, read the sports pages.

CHAPTER 35

Val's Story (Graph)

Discomfort creates growth

"I'm having a tough time staying motivated. I think I need a daily reminder or something to push me," Val said.

"I'm going to have you try something that I would NEVER tell most people to do," I offered. "And only because I know how detailed you are.

"I normally tell people to toss their weigh scales in the garbage because the average scale doesn't tell you what kind of weight you're gaining or losing. But Val, in your case, I'm going to suggest that you get a bio electric impedance scale and weigh yourself daily.

"Now here's the 'detail' part. You need to record and graph what you see each day on the scale. You're the type of person who will get motivated by seeing the changes. If you see an increase in lean mass and a decrease in body fat you will continue doing whatever you're doing. If the opposite happens, you will adjust accordingly.

"I did this for over three years with my nutrition. I recorded everything I put in my face and noted the results. This little exercise has led me to become an intuitive eater. As an example TheKim&I were out and about one day, and I just knew we had eaten too many carbs and not enough protein by the last meal of the day. So I suggested that we have two chicken breasts and a salad for dindin and no carbs. That put us right back on target for a day of perfect macro ratios."

"That sounds a little tedious," she said tentatively.

"Here's the message of hope," I said. "You don't have to get anal about the thing and do it for three years like I did. I wanted to see what absolutely everything did to my numbers. You really only need to do it for a few weeks to get a darn good idea of how your body reacts to certain foods," I assured her.

"Ok, cool. Where do I get a... you know, one of those scales?" she said with a lot more excitement.

Transferable Life Skill

People can stay motivated in different ways to do things. One way for detailed, type A people, is to measure, record and graph their results. It can provide a perfect "visual" so that, at a glance you can see your progress. This is something all successful businesses do and something that will go a long way in any life endeavor.

CHAPTER 36

Sid's Story (Incentive)

There's always a price to pay – pay it

"Hey, where did ya get the cool Marine t-shirt?" Sid asked pointing to the shirt that I was wearing when I removed my training hoodie.

I decided to indulge myself. After all, he asked. "A past client of mine moved to California a few years ago. My wife (TheKim) and I had become very good friends with them and we've kept in touch all these years. One day I got an email from him saying that her favourite band, Journey, was playing at the California Mid State Fair and we could stay at their palace overlooking the vineyards in the valley. When I told TheKim, the words had barely left my lips and she had plane tickets for us to visit.

"Anyhoo, we get to the fair and we're cruising the exhibits on the grounds when we run into a recruiting display put on by the U.S. Marines. There's a half dozen of them standing around looking buff, answering questions and promoting the lifestyle. I notice a contraption in front of the booth and ask them what they're doing with it.

"'Pull ups!' says one of the Marines. 'If you can do five pull ups we'll give you a Marine mouse pad.'

"I could barely contain myself. Ooooooo, the only good thing about that is that it has one of my favourite sayings, 'Pain is Weakness Leaving the Body!'

"The Marine was obviously not impressed by my underwhelming lack of enthusiasm so he upped the ante. 'If you can do ten pull ups, we'll give you a Marine water bottle that says the same thing.'"

"Now that's sounding a little more serious," I said.

"I think he was feeling a bit challenged coz he returned the favour and tossed in the whole enchilada and said, 'Hey, if you can do twenty pull ups I'll give you a Marine t-shirt that says, 'Pain is Weakness Leaving the Body'!'

"I looked him straight in the eyes and said, 'Let me see the shirt.' I thought to myself, 'Oh yeah, you want me to draw attention to your booth for a cheap cotton t-shirt'. But when he showed it to me, it turned out to be a high quality black Adidas style Climacool t-shirt with the Marine logo on the front and my fave saying on the back! I didn't want to tell him that I *needed* that shirt, so I just said, 'Get my t-shirt ready dude!'

"When I completed the task, the Marine tosses my shirt to me and turns to one of our crew and asks, 'How old is he?' When they told him that I was 60, he does the old double take and exclaims, 'Freakin' unbelievable!'

"We actually went back the very next day because we also had tickets to see the band Earth Wind and Fire. I decided I wanted to win a matching t-shirt for TheKim so we could wear them together. We searched the grounds high and low for those Marines but they had pulled up stakes and shipped out. They must have heard we were coming and they didn't want to give away all their goodies to that little old dude. Roger that!"

Transferable Life Skill

Sometimes you're going to be motivated by the strangest little things. It doesn't always have to be serious or for high stakes. Just get in there and have some fun. Work hard, play hard.

CHAPTER 37

Abby's Story (Belief System)

Do it or don't – no more excuses

We had just started training again for about a month after a tempo-rary layoff, and I could just tell that Abby was frustrated and disil-lusioned. Her slightly vacuous look told me that her spirit had joined Elvis and left the building. It didn't seem to be in the playground with us. Nowhere to be found.

"Abby are you ok today?" I asked.

"Yeah, why?" she asked half-heartedly as she put down her dumb-bells.

"You just don't seem to be as engaged as you normally are," I said. "Something on your mind?"

Almost in tears, she blurted, "I thought I would be a lot further ahead by now and you said last session that I wasn't putting enough effort into my cardio sessions and I don't have any more time to de-vote to my cardio and I don't think I'll ever get the results I'm working so hard for... and... "

I stepped back. "Whoa, whoa! Yes, you've been working hard. But it's only been a month. What kind of results were you expecting?"

"When we started training again, you said that I could lose two pounds a week. That's eight pounds by now and I sure haven't lost that," she fired back.

"But Abby, you didn't want to do body comps when we started up again so I can't be sure, but if you've been eating clean, along with our sessions, and with the cardio you've been doing, I'm going to say that you've probably lost fat and put on some lean mass, so your weight may not have changed that much. Have your clothes been fitting looser?" I asked.

"I don't know. You said that the cardio I was doing wasn't going to work," she continued.

"Oops. I said that because of the short period of time that you can commit to your cardio. It would be more effective to do interval, HIIT-style training. I just wanted you to raise the intensity," I explained.

"But I'm going hard. I'm sweating. I can't go harder!" she said.

"Then you're doing it right. The best you can do is the best you can do," I said. "Not to worry. You're still burning calories. If your portion controller ain't broke, at the end of the day you should still be in a caloric deficit."

"But I want results!" she demanded.

"Abby, finish this sentence for me please. Fat loss is… ?" I asked.

Immediately, without taking a breath, she responded with, "Fat loss is really hard. Especially at my age."

"Ok there's a limiting belief. Remember what Henry Ford said, 'Whether you think you can or you think you can't, you're right'," I continued. "Has anyone else your age done this? Any friends? Any one you know? If they can do it, you can do it!"

"Yeah, ok. Jennifer and Rachel did get great results," she admitted.

"Abby if it was easy, what would you do differently?" I asked.

"I don't know. I've tried everything I can," she said.

"Everything?" I asked. "What are the last twenty things you've tried?"

"Ok, ok, I'm getting it. I have to try harder," she relented.

"Maybe not 'harder'… just 'something different'. I'm totally convinced that deep down inside everybody knows how they can do one more thing, better," I said. "We have inside us the answers we need to be the very best we can be. There's got to be one small thing that you can think of. Let's make it number twenty one. If I pressed a gun to your head and told you that you had ten seconds to come up with something. What would you say?"

"I guess I would say that I CAN do this, and I'll recheck my meal portions," she said.

"Yeah, now you're talkin'! Here. Let me put the gun away!"

Transferable Life Skill

Limiting beliefs will never serve you. When you're telling yourself that you can't do something you need to stop and ask yourself if it's an excuse. Has anyone else done it? How can you do it? What else can you try? There's always an answer. Dig deep for the answer. Be unstoppable!

CHAPTER 38

Maxine's Story (Genetics)
Yesterday was the last day for excuses

It was a beautiful evening at the golf clubhouse for a great dinner with eight FUNtabulous friends. During our conversation on health and fitness Maxine just had to say, "The reason you're in such good shape is because of your genetics." I was shocked! Maxine is a pretty intelligent gal in most other ways but this tripe required a "Forrest Gump"... "stupid is as stupid does" response. So I unleashed on her. "Yeah, luckily I got the 'discipline gene' from both parents! And from that I was rewarded with diligence, self-control, persistence and focus."

Realizing her faux pas, she did the old 'Mohammed Ali back pedal'. "What I meant was... genetics will make or break you. If your parents are obese, you're going to be obese. If they're both thin, you're going to be slim as well."

"I guess I beat my genetics," I said. "You should have seen both of my parents. Neither of them were poster kids for the fitness movement!

"Here's the way to think about it. Genetics is the hand you're dealt. Yes, to a degree, it can determine your height, eye color, bone size and perhaps even your intelligence. But YOU decide on how you're going to play the hand! You can change your body composition!

"I ABSolutely love the doctor, who when told by his obese patient that, 'Obesity runs in my family,' had the intestinal fortitude to respond, 'Madam, NOBODY runs in your family!'"

I added, "Research in epigenetics and quantum physics are proving over and over again that your environment influences your genes more than you can ever know. Our genes don't determine everything.

We get to have a say in the conversation, and we can certainly control our environment in many ways."

Then Maxine asked the question of all questions. "What's the easiest way to change my body composition?"

"The easiest? NEAT!" I told her. "Non-exercise activity thermogenesis. Movement outside of the playground. Getting up and walking over to another room. Picking up your briefcase. Even fidgeting. They all contribute to your total daily calorie burn."

"Those things aren't going to help much," she said doubtfully.

I agreed. "You asked for the 'easiest' way... not the most effective or efficient way. You're right. It would take a long time to see a difference with NEAT alone. More effort, more results.

"Keep in mind, there are three kinds of movement. 'Functional movement' is walking. Some may argue this, but 'fun movement' might be golfing. There is only one type of movement that will dramatically transform your body. It's 'formal movement' and it almost always takes place in the playground!"

Transferable Life Skill

If you're going to blame irresponsible decisions on something, let it not be something you have some control over. Excuses have prevented more people from achieving their dreams and becoming the best versions of themselves than anything else, genetics included. Research is demonstrating quite convincingly that your ability to shape your own future is more within your grasp than you could ever imagine.

CHAPTER 39

Ally's Story (Events)

Don't get to the end of life and realize you only lived half of it

Ally approached the desk, waved at me and said, "I haven't made any progress for the last six months. What's going on?"

Julee, our MOD, came up & asked, "What are you two discussing?"

"Ally has plateaued again and I was about to explain a possible remedy," I answered.

"THIS... I have to hear!" Julee exclaimed.

"First you need a little background. Is it okay to share?" I asked Ally.

"Definitely," she said, not realizing that it would get rather uncomfortable.

"Julee, I've been working with Ally for the last twelve years or so, writing programs and providing nutrition guidance, but she wasn't really ready to make the changes I suggested. Until about three years ago.

"Unfortunately in order to make a change, whether that's to initiate a health program, or to get off a plateau, a person needs to have good reasons. Sometimes that takes an 'event'. Now hopefully it's not a catastrophic 'event' like a heart attack, where they realize at the worst possible moment that they should have taken better care of themselves. It's always better to 'witness' someone else's 'event', where they can look on and say, 'I'm going to start taking better care of myself so that doesn't happen to me'.

"The better way to go is to have what I call a 'mini event'. Maybe they take a few pictures of themselves and see if the images are what they actually thought they looked like. Sometimes that just may be enough to kick start a great fitness and nutrition plan.

"I remember when the four year old grandson of one of my client's catapulted him into our beautiful relationship when he pointed to Grandpa's porcine belly and said, 'Gee Grandpa, you sure got a lot of food in there!'

"Another 'mini event' would be to 'self-impose' an 'event'... such as signing up for a half marathon. THAT will get a person going. And that is exactly what Ally did three years ago. And boy, did she get in shape! Lost a ton of fat and increased her endurance at least ten-fold! FUNtabulous job!" I said as I opened my arms to 'present' Ally.

Ally looked on and smiled with pride. "Yep, that was a really great year! But now I need to progress again."

"Ok, sorry Ally, but here's where it gets a bit uncomfy... you said I could share. You're resting on your past laurels. You're in good shape and you know it. You also know how much work it takes to get there. AND the crazy amount of work to go further yet. But all the suggestions I've made in the last couple of months have gone in one ear and out the other, just like they did those first years we trained before you were ready to really get after it."

Ally turned a little red and nodded sheepishly.

"You're going to need some really good reasons to step up your game, or perhaps, you need an event!" I added. "Until you do, things will remain just the way they are!"

Transferable Life Skill

I remember hearing Diana Ross explain what the "grade C" meant. I will paraphrase. It meant... "Cheat! You cheated yourself and all the world of what you could have done, and failed to make your full contribution." It's easy to look at your situation and compare it to others less praiseworthy. But if you decide not to do the best you can do, you've cheated.

Find your reasons or create an event, something that propels you forward to a whole new level! Life is not a practice run!

CHAPTER 40

Mel's Story (Faith)

You are ON the way or IN the way

As I toured the exercise floor I approached Mel on her elliptical trainer. I could tell that something was not quite right. She didn't look like her usual happy upbeat self.

"Howz you doin' Mel?" I asked.

She stated bluntly, "Good."

"Really? You should notify your face. You just don't look like a happy camper," I said. "What's really going on?"

I'm just not seeing any results," she said sadly.

"Mel, it's only been a month!" I exclaimed.

"But shouldn't something have happened by now?" she whined.

"Last week when I saw you, I thought you said that you've lost six pounds?" I reminded her.

Sarcastically she said, "Oh wow, I've only got 44 more to go."

"C'mon. How long did it take you to put on the weight?" I said. "And it's supposed to melt off in a month?"

"Well, yeah… I guess," she stammered.

I decided to shoot the works. "Mel, the captain of a ship can't see his destination for fully 99 per cent of his trip. But he most certainly knows that if he stays the course and follows his maps and instruments, that barring unforeseen calamities, he will arrive at his port at the expected time. Even if a storm takes him off course he knows how to correct it and get back on it if he follows the plan."

"Ok, I'll just keep following the plan. I guess something is working," she admitted.

"Keep it up and you'll nail the goal before Christmas!" I assured her.

Transferable Life Skill

Don't give up. Don't let fear take you off course. Fear and faith both require that you believe in something you can't see. Always choose faith - believe in the plan.

CHAPTER 41

Adison's Story (Prep)

Growth not comfort

"Sometimes I just can't get started. I know I want to run in the morning, and I plan for it, but that old bed is so darn warm and comfy. Got any good ideas?" Adison asked.

I thought for a moment. "When you say that you plan for your run in the morning, how are you doing that?"

She said, "I put it in my calendar."

"Do you tell the family that you're not going to be available at that time?"

"Yep, they know."

"How often have you missed your run this year?"

"Only a half dozen times."

"That's not too bad. Howz 'bout this? Put your running gear right next to your bed so that everything is ready to go and you don't have to go looking for it. Alarm goes off. Jump into your stuff and you're out the door!" I suggested.

"But sometimes I just hit the snooze button," she admitted.

"Hitting the snooze button puts you behind the power curve right off the bat! I didn't want to do this to you, but now we bring out the big guns. If you're gonna be like that... put your alarm clock on the dresser across the room. Get a couple of cookie tins and put them right beside your bed, where you would step on to the floor as you throw back the covers when you get up. Now get a pitcher of water and pour some into each cookie tin. Voila! That's called morning enticement."

Transferable Life Skill

There are times when extreme measures are called for. If other strategies don't work, get creative and have fun.

CHAPTER 42

Reena's Story (Environment)

Don't give away your power

I could tell that Reena was a little off when she strolled in for our session. She had a faraway look in her eyes and she wasn't fully present so I asked her, "Something bothering you today?"

"Why do you ask?"

"You're just not as focused as usual and we're starting your new program today. So in order to avoid an accident and an ambulance ride home we should figure out why you're having trouble concentrating."

She broke down. "Ok look. I'm not getting any support from my friends, or even at home. Here I am taking care of my health and everyone makes me feel guilty when I come to the gym to work out, as if I abandoned them and I'm just being selfish."

I started with a little levity. "First, this is our playground, not a gym. And second, Reena, there will be times when some people, even those who love us, will not be ready to stand behind us in all our endeavors.

"The health and fitness journey is not one that most people take even though deep down they know they should. Some people feel guilty when they see you doing something that they know they should be doing for themselves, but can't find the discipline to do. So in order to feel better about themselves, they need to bring you down to their level and get you to stop."

She replied, "But if they truly cared about me, surely they would want me to take care of my health. Wouldn't they?"

"Yes. And I'm sure that they do care about you and want you to be healthy, but they also notice you feeling and looking better and better all the time. And it's difficult for them to admit that they don't have the same drive or discipline that you have. Sometimes they're just jealous."

"So what do I do?"

"Your environment is very important. You should always surround yourself with the kind of people that you would like to be. Do they have their priorities right? Do they really care about you? Can they support you?" I added.

"But some of these people are family! Even my own husband is questioning me!" she said.

"Ok, the first thing I would do is explain to them how important it is to you to continue your healthy lifestyle. Tell them all the benefits you're getting. Let them know that you're not going to stop and then invite them to come with you. Sometimes people will go with someone else but they won't go on their own, and having a workout buddy is a huge bonus."

"What if they won't join me?"

"You can't force them to come to the playground, just as you can't force them to quit trying to make you feel guilty. You can however, tell them that when they start criticizing you, you will point both fingers to the sides of your head and inform them that 'these are ears, not garbage cans', and to make no mistake... they will be tuned out."

She pushed further. "And if that doesn't work?"

"Geez Reena, you got a tough crowd there! Sorry but there comes a time when you have to make choices. Bless them and go on to the next. Only surround yourself with supportive people who truly care about you."

"Alright, done. But what about my spouse?"

"I'm not going there! A good heart-to-heart... or perhaps some couples counselling? This one is out of my scope of practice. But... you sold him once! You can sell him again!"

Transferable Life Skill

Many very successful people were laughed at and ridiculed until they proved that they knew what they were doing. If you're doing the right thing, sometimes you will have to make tough decisions. Your environment... the people you associate with should always be the kind of people that you admire and respect. Remember, there are typically three conversations going on in any social gathering. In one corner they're talking about other people... LEAVE that conversation. In another corner, they're talking about events... do not linger. The place you really want to be... you need to be... is in the corner where they're talking about IDEAS! Ideas on how to become the very best you can be... life changing ideas!

There are three-minute people, three-hour people and three-day people. Remember, the time you spend, you will never get back! Decide and make it count!

CHAPTER 43

Alisha's Story (Commitment)

Winners do the little things that failures don't like to do

Alisha was a referral from Craig. He asked me if she could contact me regarding a few training questions.

The alarm went off immediately when we met the very first time. "Hi Randy. I've been told that you can get me down to eight percent body fat," she said.

Now you had to see Alisha. She was about 5'8" and 134 pounds. And as I was later to discover... 24 per cent body fat.

"Yep I can. But I won't," I told her.

She looked at me strangely. "What? Why not?"

"Eight per cent body fat is way too low for an adult female," I said. "And at the expense of encouraging a harassment charge, if you don't mind me saying, you look great just as you are. Most women would kill to look like you."

"Ok I'll come clean with you. We're having a transformation contest at my office and I intend to win no matter what," she admitted.

Now I've heard these kinda folks before (they're very rare) and if there's one thing I love, it's determination and dedication, so I just had to test her.

"Alisha, do you actually know what kind of ordeal you're about to thrust upon yourself?"

"How hard can it be? I see people in the gym every day who look really great," she continued.

"Yep, they do. What you may not be aware of is the extra hard work and sacrifices that fitness models and bodybuilders make in order to compete. The attention to detail regarding calorie and water intake, macro nutrient ratios and training schedules is absurd. Discipline is a huge factor. Then there's the deprivation, cutting carbs and calories, eliminating sweets, most of their favorite meals and later sodium. Their social lives can really suck unless they hang with other competitors. They can get hungry, moody and dehydrated. And eight percent body fat will screw up your cycles. Sound good?" I cautioned.

"I'm ready for it!" she assured me.

Wow, this girl either had incredible drive or her prefrontal lobe had a severe misfire. "Here's the deal breaker, and I'm going to take you at your word on this. You ABSolutely have to promise me that when I take you to eight percent body fat for the contest, immediately after it's over, you will re-feed and back off the transformation training. I want to see you back to your normal healthy body fat within two weeks. Are we on the same page?"

"Done," she promised.

So I did. She did. She won her contest and was back to 22 per cent body fat soon after.

Transferable Life Skill

Ask yourself the hard questions before you embark on the journey. Learn what it's going to take to be successful and then decide if it is, in fact, for you. You must be fully aware, going in. Are you prepared to do the hard work? If so, do it with conviction!

CHAPTER 44

Jordan's Story (Motivation)
Motivate the mind – the body will follow

"I need an energy infusion," Jordan informed me as he shuffled into the playground.

At the expense of sounding dispassionate, I smiled and said, "Awww, what's the problem Jordie?"

"Man, I gotta tell ya, I'm feeling too tired to work out today," he admitted.

"Well the beautiful thing is, and it's a testimony to your dedication, you managed to crawl in here. And on time I might add," I assured him.

"Yeah, but it's hard to find the energy sometimes," he added.

"I've always believed that you find the energy to do the things that you want to do, your priorities, your values. Everybody has way more energy than they wish to admit," I said.

"Here let me give you an example. Let's say that you're at home lying on your couch. All of a sudden you hear your garage door open. Now you know that nobody is leaving and nobody is expected, so I think you're going to find the energy to get up and hunt down the invader. Or here's another. You're lying on that same couch watching the vacuum tube. You see a commercial for something and you realize, 'Uh oh, I've got a date tonight that requires one of those. Time to get off the couch and get moving.' Or here's one. You're giving that same couch another good workout and the doorbell rings. It's an old buddy you haven't seen in years. He's in town and wants to go for a coffee and catch up. I think you're pumped and ready to go. Would I be right?" I asked.

He agreed. "But what do I do if my buddy doesn't show and I want to lie there instead of working out?"

"Well first, burn the damn couch. Then use that beautiful faculty that separates us from the rest of the animals on the planet, imagination! Just imagine how great you're going to feel after the workout... the endorphins... the serotonin... the dopamine... the adrenaline... the circulation boost... that nice clear mind... and ultimately... the physical results."

"Sometimes I just can't think like that, you know. I can't be bothered," he said.

"Now that's troubling," I said. "That's 'reward motivation'. Maybe that particular day it won't make you move. Maybe that day you're gonna need 'fear motivation'," I offered.

"That doesn't sound good. What's that?"

"You again, use your miraculous imagination. But this time, you project yourself 25 years into the future. Use the 'rocking chair technique'. And this time ask yourself, 'what does my health look like after all those skipped work outs? How functional am I? Can I do all the things with my grandkids that I'd like to do? Am I as independent as I want to be? What if I had just had more discipline?'" I added.

"Yikes!" Jordan exclaimed. "That's kinda rough, isn't it?"

"Something's gotta get you off the couch man. And if reward and fear don't do it, the third type of motivation is most certainly not in the plan.

"Ok, what's the third type?"

"The third kind of motivation is 'attitude motivation'. You will have explored both the rewards and the fears, a kind of cost/benefit analysis, and you have actually changed your attitude about your actions. Ideally and ultimately, this is where you want to be because you encounter the least conflict and procrastination. It's a no brainer. You've become a Nike commercial. You 'Just Do It!'"

Transferable Life Skill

Napoleon Hill said that the imagination is the most inconceivably powerful force the world has ever known, and we all have one working for us whenever we want. He also writes about the transmission of energy. Take the energy that you would be using for something unproductive and transmute it into a positive fruitful activity that will bode well for your future and help you become the best you can be. Use whichever of the three types of motivation that will help you get the job done.

CHAPTER 45

Ina's Story (Macro/Micro)
Be an elite mental performer

"Hey Gymja... how's things going?" I asked my favorite little playground amazon warrior as she appeared to be resting against a stability ball, propped against the wall in the playground.

Ina looked up at me. "This wall sit exercise that one of the trainers gave me is not that hard. I can do it for over three minutes," she bragged.

"Hmmm... maybe if you did it right," I laughed. "You'd find it more challenging."

She demonstrated her best form. "What's wrong with this?" she asked.

"Well if I took a picture of you from the side, I think you'd see that your legs are not even close to a 90 degree angle, maybe 120 degrees at best. You're standing way too erect to get anything out of the exercise," I said.

She looked puzzled. "I don't get it."

"Look Gymja, think extremes. Think of it this way. Micro/macro. If you were to stand straight up and lean on the ball, one extreme (micro), you wouldn't feel anything in your quads would you?"

"I guess not," she said as she tried it.

"Now try the exercise with your bottom as close to the floor as you can. This is the other extreme (macro). Any difference?" I asked.

"Oooh yeah!" she cried as her legs started shaking beneath her. "That's way better!"

Transferable Life Skill

A great way to compare most ideas, techniques or strategies is to think in the extremes - micro/macro. The answer to the question of which is better should become apparent as you explore the concept. It will also help to combine this method with a "Ben Franklin". He would draw a vertical line down the middle of a page of paper and make a list of "pros" and "cons" and look for the column with the most entries. This can be refined by "weighing" the entries ie. a "soft pro" such as... "the candy dish is closer than the fruit bowl"... versus a "hard con" such as... "the sugar content in the candy"... when making a treat decision. This will most definitely fine tune the process.

CHAPTER 46

Kim Anne's Story (Mental Modelling)

You don't get what you deserve – you get what you expect

"OMG! Are you alright?" Kim Anne asked as she watched me do my very best bird imitation when the front wheel of my Trikke got caught between the sidewalk and the grass. The Trikke went down hard and I continued in a forward motion over the handle bars.

"Oh yeah. I meant to do that," I kidded her as I picked up the unit and checked it over for damage.

"Wow. That was pretty impressive," she said. "Most people would have gone down and broken a wrist or an arm. But you just landed on your feet."

"In my mind, I've already gone over what I would do if I lost traction or jammed a wheel, like what just happened," I explained. "You always want to be prepared for the unexpected. And if you've drilled it over and over, your chances of a successful outcome are infinitely better.

Transferable Life Skill

Beware of the "cognitive tunnel", resting on laurels and living in the land of "Oblivion". Mental modelling for all the situations that could happen is imperative. NEVER be caught by surprise!

My wife and I have a favorite restaurant that unfortunately has their parking lot in the middle of a dark alley. When we exit the restaurant, I always make sure that she walks between me and the wall of the building. One night she was talking to me but I was focused on the sole light behind a dumpster we were passing. She immediately berated me. "You're not listening to me. What are you looking at?"

I told her that I was watching for shadows or movement behind the dumpster.

She then told me, "You're so weird. Why do you think like that?"

At which point I explained to her that someday she might be very happy that I thought "like that" and proceeded to explain cognitive tunnels versus mental mapping.

PART 2

30% Nutrition

Yes, this is a huge part of the equation. But certainly not 80 per cent worth like a lot of people would have you believe.

And again, it's simple but it's not easy.

I have found that the transformation journey can be more difficult if a person is a "foodie" because they get bored easily without variety in their menus. The transformation winners who could eat the same perfectly balanced meals day in and day out always got the best results.

I'm not, at all, saying that you have to adopt a boring diet, but it certainly helps if you don't consider food to be your reason for being. Eat to live. DO NOT live to eat.

Therefore, this may be part of the psychological factor, in that, when you overcome your cravings for different foods, you're on your way to a quicker more permanent transformation. The following chapters will help you understand nutrition and eliminate cravings.

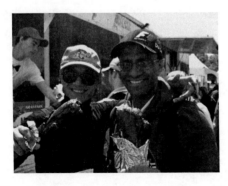

Dr. J and I enjoying some FI protein

Photo by random bum with a crappy old iPhone – M. Yan

CHAPTER 47

Barb's Story (Macros)

I think – feel – and perform as a champion

"How much protein?" she said rather loudly.

"Your macro nutrient ratio will be 40/40/20. We're shooting for 40 per cent of your diet in protein, 40 per cent carbs and 20 per cent healthy fats.

"Look," I said. "I know it sounds like a lot. And I know that registered dieticians have always had an issue with trainers and fitness competitors for their protein prescriptions. But really, if you want to get the results you're aiming for, you need to repair the muscle tissue that you're tearing down in the playground."

"But I've heard that too much protein will cause kidney failure," she objected.

"Not true. Kidney transplants do not run rampant among fitness competitors. Also, just for insurance, we prescribe a lot of water so that you can flush those puppies out."

"So what are good sources of protein?" she queried.

"The bodybuilder's staples are chicken breasts, tuna and egg whites. You can't go wrong following the most knowledgeable people when it comes to transforming their bodies."

"But won't it get boring eating chicken every day?"

"Yep, I remember when Porter Freeman, a division winner in the very first Body for Life Contest said, in his beautiful southern accent, 'If I ate another chicken breast I was going to start growing feathers and pecking gravel.'

"What are you prepared to do to achieve your goal?"

Transferable Life Skill

There will be times when you need to ignore some "experts" and rely on "what works".

CHAPTER 48

Stacy's Story (Quick Fixes)
To get past it – you gotta go through it

After only six months of training, Stacy said, "I'm getting liposuction!"

"Otay. But you DO know how lipo works, right?" I asked.

"Well, sorta," she replied.

"They suck out a bunch of fat cells from your trouble area. Those fat cells are gone. They can never give you problems again. Here's where it gets ugly. IF you don't change your lifestyle(which most people don't) meaning that they were taking in more calories than they were burning off before the lipo to accumulate excess fat in the first place, and after lipo, they're still gorging out and still not moving enough. Those excess calories have to go somewhere. So the fat gets stored in other fat cells, the cells that were left behind. No more jiggly under arms but now your thighs become the problem."

"Well how about that doctor who advertises on the radio?" she asked.

"That's dangerous as all get out. Don't do that! I've heard from a lot of people who've done it. They said that they were restricted to approximately 700 hundred calories per day. ANYBODY will lose weight on 700 hundred calories. The problem is threefold:

"One, NOBODY can get enough micro nutrients. That's vitamins and minerals, on 700 hundred calories a day. So patients are 'invited' to go into the clinic regularly for a syringe full of vitamins. Shot straight into the belly! Fun times! Especially if you love needles!

"Two, NOBODY can live off 700 hundred calories forever. It's unsustainable!

"And three, on 700 hundred calories what kind of weight are you losing? It'll be water, fat and muscle. NOT good! Muscle is your metabolic engine. When you go off the diet and start eating normally, with your decreased metabolism, you end up putting on more weight than you dropped! This is the very definition of 'yo-yo dieting'!"

Not giving up, she added, "Has there been any success with that method?"

"Only one person out of the dozen or so that I know of has managed to keep the weight off. And that one person DID change their eating and exercise habits.

"People are always looking for the 'magic pill' the 'silver bullet'! Why not just change your eating and exercise habits first and avoid the expense, the yo-yoing, and the discomfort of injections?

"Do it naturally and create a healthy lifestyle that you can count on for all the rest of your days."

Transferable Life Skill

The "quick fix" is very enticing in life. But it's almost never worth it. There's nothing worse than getting temporary results and then having to start over from a negative starting point. Remember the first major Law of the Universe… the Law of Cause and Effect - what you put in is what you get out.

CHAPTER 49

Meagan's Story (Sups)
Make sure you do all you can do

"Should I take supplements? Do you take any sups?" Meagan asked as I finished writing up her nutrition plan.

"Yep, I take vitamin D, omega 3 and a multi every day."

"But I've read that it's all just a waste of money and that you're just creating expensive pee," she countered.

"Well the way I look at it, is that NO one can get perfectly balanced meals 100 per cent of the time. So it's just cheap insurance and I'm not really sure those 'bioavailability' claims made by some companies are not just a lot of propaganda to sell product.

"I actually went to a meeting where a company was demonstrating how their product was so much more 'bio available' than another. They dropped both products into a clear glass of water on the stage and told us to watch what happened. Their pill dissolved in the water but the other pill remained in its original form. It was pretty convincing, except for one thing. The stomach uses acid not water, to digest material. So I'm thinking that both products would be bio available... not just the expensive one that they were trying to push!"

Transferable Life Skill

Sometimes you just need a little outside help. Don't be afraid to ask for it... when you need it.

CHAPTER 50

Roxanna's Story (Skipping Meals)

Energy – You can't give whatchoo don't got

She was sitting on the edge of the weight bench, her face pale and her body slightly shaking. This was not her typical condition after only a half hour into her session so I asked, "Roxanna, what have you had to eat today?"

"Two carrots and an apple," came the weak reply.

"Look, I know you want to lose body fat but this is not the way to do it. You need energy to get through your workouts and you can't let your blood sugar drop to this degree," I said.

"But it doesn't make sense. You always said 'calories in/calories out'."

"I know this is going to sound counter intuitive but when you're training hard, especially to gain lean mass, you need to eat MORE than you're probably used to eating... not less... and right now you're running outta gas. You're not gonna make it to the podium."

I implored her. "For our next session, please promise me that you'll get more calories?"

"That's for sure," she puffed.

Transferable Life Skill

Sometimes you just need to have faith in what works. It may not seem logical but if others have proven it works, it could work for you as well. Read the signals.

CHAPTER 51

Barbie's Story (Carbs)
What you want to be tomorrow – you gotta do today

Barbie was dejected as she looked at her fat loss results on her weekly body composition analysis. "Should I stop eating carbs?"

"That's fairly controversial," I said. "A lot of people think they should eliminate carbs from their diet in order to lose weight. But I have to tell you that balance is the name of the game. You're training regularly so some carbs are your friends."

"But I know someone who dumped the carbs and she lost a bunch of weight. I think it was the Keto diet."

"Yep... look, I won't bash any particular diet," I replied. "I bash ALL diets. I'm not a big fan of diets. They all work in the beginning coz they're typically calorie reduced. But the main problem is that they're just not sustainable.

"I believe that we should all be on a balanced clean eating plan that contains the right amount of calories for our daily energy expenditure. No diets, just a lifelong healthy nutrition strategy."

"I know you hate this," she pleaded. "But I just want to get some quick results."

"Otay. Look Barbie let's try something less harsh. Why not try eliminating some of your starchy carbs?"

"What are those?"

"Those are carbs that you CAN do without... potatoes, rice, bread, pasta... save them for cheat day unless you're running a marathon.

"At the very least, if you want to play with carbs we could try carb tapering... have the majority of your carbs at the very beginning of your day and slowly eliminate them until your last meal... then, no carbs."

"That might be do-able."

"The other strategy you might try is carb cycling. Cardio day would be a higher carb day to replace glycogen... perhaps 50 per cent of your diet in healthy low glycemic, complex carbs. Resistance day would be higher protein to repair tissue... with perhaps 25 per cent carbs."

"Yeah, I could do that too."

Transferable Life Skill

Extremes are not your friends. Balance is better, but sometimes you can modify the equation for quicker results. Don't be afraid to experiment, provided you don't leave any important components out of the mix. Always aim for sustainability. Experiment to see what works for you.

CHAPTER 52

Amanda's Story (Sugar Cravings)

Excellence never comes easy

"My sweet tooth is really getting the best of me!" Amanda stated. "What can I do?"

I nodded in agreement. "Yep, I hear ya. My sweet tooth used to run rough shod over my best intentions as well. I would be returning home and almost be in the garage when I'd turn the car around and drive all the way to the store I just passed to buy a bag of sour berry candies. Sometimes a pound at a time... and then polish them all off on the way home! Darn good thing I'm so freakin' active. I wasn't gaining any weight but at one point I realized that this was not a good thing! These sugar carbs were going to kill me eventually."

Amanda laughed. "Well hello Mr. Trainer. Glad to see that you're human after all."

"Oh believe me, I'm all too human. Just ask my wife," I continued. "So this is how I got out of the habit. First I made sure that I learned what carbs really are and how they affected my body.

"If you look at a complex carb under a microscope you'll see a long sugar chain. If you look at a simple carb under a microscope you'll see a short sugar chain. Either way they both cause your pancreas to up-regulate your insulin levels... and insulin is a fat storing hormone.

"Not even diet pop was going to work! The artificial sweetener spiked insulin just as much as the sugar and still created a dopamine hit that causes a craving for more. Man I just couldn't win!"

Amanda agreed. "That's the way I'm feeling!"

"But knowing that cancer cells love sugar and that it creates abdominal fat which contributes to diabetes, heart conditions, cancers and all kinds of ugly things, I slowly weaned myself off the white stuff. Visceral fat is NOT your friend."

She said, "Cold turkey?"

"I still have sour berries a couple of times a year. But usually when I get that craving I turn to the fridge which has a bowl of washed grapes, apples, oranges, baby carrots, snap peas, cherries and baby tomatoes to satisfy that sweet tooth.

"Wean yourself off the bad stuff and make substitutions. Not easy but very do-able and highly rewarding! You will be very surprised at how much quicker you achieve your results!

"You know Bob, right?" I asked.

"Oh yeah, I talk to him when he's on the stationary bike quite often," she said.

"Next time you see him, ask him how he lost 25 pounds in six months by doing nothing extra but cutting out sugar!"

Transferable Life Skill

Think deeply about how a bad habit is *really* affecting you. What are the true repercussions? Learn everything you can about the culprit. Then every time you find yourself gravitating in that direction, ask yourself if the outcome is what you truly want. Find substitutes.

CHAPTER 53

Ann's Story (Wine)
If nothing changes – nothing changes

As we sat down to set up her nutrition plan, Ann gave me the stink eye and stated, "I'll follow your nutrition plan, but I am NOT giving up my wine!"

I nodded. "You know that a protein is four calories per gram. A carbohydrate is four calories per gram. And a fat is nine calories per gram. Ann, alcohol is seven empty calories per gram. Are you sure you won't moderate the wine?"

"Oh, I'm very sure!" she said emphatically.

"Otay, then howzbout we make it into a food group? Let's incorporate it into your carb allocation. If you take a good multi vitamin and you can maintain your energy for training we'll test drive this for a week or so to see the results. Fair nuff?"

"Done!"

Well... wine allocation didn't work for Ann. We eventually had to wean her down to half of her usual intake.

Transferable Life Skill

It's ok to try to fool yourself. After all, if you can't fool yourself, who can you fool? But when the "self-regulating" plan doesn't work, it's time to get real and do what you knew you should have done all along. Self-discipline is your friend!

CHAPTER 54

Vera's Story (Chocolate)

Engage in the practice of self-mastery

Another "before and after" picture I show to new clients is Vera. She lost 20 pounds and eleven and three quarter inches in the 12 week program. She was tickled pink with her results but at the end she confessed. "I think I could have done a better job but I'm a chocoholic and I indulged a few times too often."

I was shocked. "Vera, why didn't you tell me that you had a chocolate addiction? I could have given you some strategies to beat it."

"What would you have told me?" she asked.

"I would have suggested that possibly you could have taken a good meal replacement bar, cut it up into pieces and had a couple for a quick fix."

"That might have worked."

I followed up. "And remember. Protein is your friend when it comes to staving off cravings because it stabilizes blood sugar as well as keeping you full longer. Also, the thermic effect of protein is considerably higher than that of a carb or a fat. In other words, roughly 30 per cent of the calories in a protein are required just to digest it. A carb requires 15 per cent to 20 per cent and a fat requires around two per cent to three per cent. So your net caloric intake from a protein is only 70 per cent as opposed to 97 to 98 per cent with a fat."

She thought for a second. "I think it might be the fat in the chocolate that I need."

"Omega fats will keep you full and help you stave off cravings as well. But you can get too much of a good thing. Remember that all fats, omegas included, are still nine calories per gram versus the four calories per gram in a protein. So when the smoke clears, you could have twice the protein instead of the fat."

She admitted. "That's true for me. If I have more protein and fat when I'm dining out at a restaurant I very often don't need dessert."

"Yep, let me give you a couple of other restaurant tips: When you place your order always ask your server to ONLY serve you half and put the other half in a puppy sack."

"Gee, I get a nice meal the next day too!" she said.

"Bonus! Another great idea is to play the 'dip and stab'. Always order salad dressing 'on the side' and instead of pouring it all over your salad, dip your fork in the dressing and then stab your salad. You'll be pleasantly surprized to see all the dressing you have left over, as opposed to having a bowl swimming in it when you're done."

"Hey, great idea!"

"One last trick. Always down a 10 ounce glass of good ol' H20 before you fire anything into your mouth. It'll fill you up a bit... cause you to eat less and it'll contribute to your daily water intake."

Transferable Life Skill

Rather than keeping "secrets" from your master mind group, share what you're feeling or going through, and in most cases, they can help you overcome the challenges. After all, that's the reason they're there. Communication is a good thing!

CHAPTER 55

Jamie's Story (Hunger)

Go the extra mile – it's never crowded there

Rubbing his stomach just before our session, Jamie said, "I seem to be hungry all the time. What gives?"

"Here's a great trick. I once read a doctor's suggestion to drink a 10 ounce glass of water anytime you feel hungry. Wait 10 minutes. And if you're still hungry reach for a healthy snack. He said that very often people confuse dehydration with the feeling of hunger. They're not really hungry. They're just thirsty.

"Also, make sure that you're getting the prescribed amount of protein and omega fats. They'll help you stave off hunger.

"Now having said that, Veronica, one of our members said something that I've always remembered and thought was brilliant. She said, 'In North America, what's wrong with being a little hungry every once in a while?'

"Kind of a first world problem I'd say?" I added.

Transferable Life Skill

Sometimes you just need to stop what you're doing for a moment and take a break or at least a deep breath and ask yourself what is really going on. Is it what you think it is or is it something altogether different and how does it affect your goal? Then try some techniques that are known to address the issue. Perspective is a good thing!

CHAPTER 56

Jacqui's Story (Cruise)

It's not okay to make excuses

"I put on seven pounds on my cruise. How could that be?" a very nicely tanned Jacqui sobbed.

"Oh come on. You had fun didn't you?" I countered. "That's what holidays are for... having fun and twisting off. Life is meant to be lived."

"Yeah but I'm not so sure it was worth it," she moaned, looking at her post-holiday body comp results.

"That's only 25 thousand calories you took in but didn't burn off," I said.

I think she started crying.

"It's kinda the same thing that happens with retired professional athletes and bodybuilders. If, after their active careers, they continue eating as if they were still training hard, they end up gaining weight and they don't look anything like they did at their peak," I explained.

"Yeah I've seen them. Muscle turns into fat so quickly," she stated.

Knowing Jacqui, I looked at her, horrified and said, "That sounds like something a sofa spud would say. Spuds don't and won't exercise. So they come up with all kinds of stupid pathetic insane excuses not to.

"Fat and muscle are two totally different types of cells. You can't turn muscle into fat any more than you can turn an eye into a nose. The problem is when an athlete reduces their training volume, but continues to eat the same way, their metabolism is slower due to muscle loss and the excess calories are stored as fat, making it look like their muscle turned into fat."

Transferable Life Skill

Always take responsibility for your situation. Going overboard every once in a while is okay but keep it to a minimum and certainly don't make silly excuses. And when the wheels fall off the bus, just put them back on and get back on the road.

CHAPTER 57

Jill's Story (Hydration)

The difference between who you are and who you want to be is what you do

I'm a stickler for clients to hydrate between sets in the playground. People don't usually get enough water as it is, but it's particularly important during a training session to replace lost fluids.

It's come to the point that some of my clients have actually started to hide their water bottles under the work out benches. Sometimes they may come clean and tell me that their back teeth are floating and they'll blow up if they swallow another drop. Or some people will attempt an explanation. This was the case with Jill. "I know I need more water but I just don't like the taste!"

"Really? What does your water taste like?" I asked.

"That's the point I guess. It doesn't," she said. "I'd like to have some flavor. How about fruit juice instead?"

"Yikes! If you came over to my house for a visit and I offered you four oranges. What would you say?" I asked.

"I don't think so. No thanks," she replied. "That's way too many."

"Good thinking. A 500ml glass of orange juice is over 200 calories. Have the orange instead. There are only a quarter of the calories in an orange.

"Now having said that, I used to think the exact same thought - water is so boring," I admitted. "But after trying different flavourings, powders, and even fruit and veggie infusions, I was able to wean myself off of any additives and go to straight water. Try to stay clear of the extra sugars and the artificial colorings. Water is the elixir of life. Your taste buds will change and they will thank you for it."

I caught her glance at her water bottle, and I smiled. "So that's why you haven't finished your water?" I asked.

She nodded.

"Jill, there are three goals when you come into the playground. One - get through Randy's stinkin' program. Two - get 'personal bests' as often as possible. And three - finish your entire water bottle!"

She grabbed her bottle. Tossed it back and finished the entire thing.

"Great job! Between your great progressions today and your water intake, you have just delayed your walker delivery by another six months!" I congratulated her.

Transferable Life Skill

When you know that you should be doing something more productive than you are, even though you find it boring or distasteful, get creative and find a different way to do it. Then give it a chance to work. You may be pleasantly surprised at how you can change for the better.

CHAPTER 58

Candice's Story (MRP)
Recalibrate

"Wanna try this new meal replacement drink I brought along?" Candice asked as she pulled a package from her suitcase. My little sister was staying at our house for the weekend to celebrate a milestone birthday. "It's banana flavoured," she added.

"Hey! Ya had me at meal replacement," I told her. "I love to test drive anything that makes our health and fitness journey more efficient, and anything other than the standard chocolate, vanilla and strawberry works for me. Bring it!"

After mixing the powder into a glass of water, she passed it to me and waited for my reaction.

"Wow! This is Pamfastic! Where's that bag? Let's see what's in it!" I said as I started to read the nutrition info. "Oopsies! Cand this is not a meal replacement shake."

"What is it?" she asked.

"It's a protein drink," I informed her.

"What's the difference?" she asked.

"A meal replacement shake has all the main macro nutrients... protein, carbohydrates and fats. Plus it has micronutrients as well," I said.

"What are micronutrients?" she asked with obvious disappointment.

"Micros are minerals and vitamins, just like you'd get if you're consuming a full whole meal."

"So what is this if it's not a meal replacement?"

"It's a protein supplement."

"What's wrong with that?"

"Nothing. If you've already had your meal and you just need to top up the protein portion. But if you 're using it to replace a meal it needs a lot more nutrients to fill the bill."

"But it says right on the back that it has all those vitamins and minerals. Look," she argued.

"Well there's the marketing trick. Yes, the nutrition label lists all the vitamins and minerals. But if you follow each item to the end of the line it shows zeroes for all of them. These people are hoping that you're not very detailed and will stop reading after you see the list of nutrients and that you won't read to the end and see that there actually isn't any in the product."

"Those creeps!" she cried.

Transferable Life Skill

Be darn sure that what you're getting is what you think it is and what you bargained for. Don't be fooled by fancy marketing or by people misrepresenting themselves or their products. Always dig a bit deeper to make sure that there are no surprises at the end of the day.

CHAPTER 59

Brandi's Story (Maintenance Nutrition)

Once you see results it becomes an addiction

I have a beautiful "niece in law" who has won many beauty contests. One of which was for her entire state in 2012, and qualified her for Miss USA.

We were having lunch one day at TheKim's Highlevel Diner when I asked her, "Brandi, now that we're relatives would it be okay to ask you a personal question?"

"Of course. We're family," she said.

I continued. "Thanks. As a personal trainer, nutrition is a huge subject for me, my clients and members. Now that you're no longer competing, what is your personal nutrition protocol?"

"I eat whatever I want," she offered.

Almost choking on my water, I stared at her and asked, "Whaaaaaa?"

"I eat whatever I want... but... I don't eat as much as I want!" she explained.

"Great strategy!" I said, as I made a mental note to pay very close attention to what she ordered. This should be really interesting I thought to myself.

When the time came to order, I could not believe what I was hearing and seeing. Brandi ordered the famous grilled chicken cheddar sandwich! A heart attack on a plate. But being the polite observer, I didn't say a word and continued to watch.

Imagine my surprise when she took only one quarter of the entire sandwich and passed the rest on for other family members at the table to try.

She's gonna starve, I thought to myself. No wonder she's still so slim and could very easily enter another competition at any time.

Now she did in fact have a salad, but what happened next, all but freaked me out. She ordered the World Famous Highlevel Diner bread pudding... WITH... the killer caramel bourbon sauce!!! I thought... REALLY? THIS I gotta see!

When the decadent desert arrived at our table, Brandi proceeded to extract one spoonful and, you guessed it, passed the rest on. Unbelievable!

"Wow! You got a turbo charged portion controller! UROCK!" I told her.

Transferable Life Skill

Exercising discipline and delaying gratification can be a very useful tool. Very often you don't need as much as you think you do. That can be food, money, love, or any number of commodities. Restricting indulgences to more reasonable amounts can be very manageable and very rewarding in the long term.

CHAPTER 60

Jake's Story (Ferraris)
No one's gonna do it for you

Between sets of heavy sit squats in our playground, Jake thoughtfully sighed. "It's really hard to establish exercise as a lifestyle with things happening all around us every day. But I really want my boys to make it a priority."

Jake and I went back a long way together and our greatest common interest was Formula One racing and performance cars in general. So I thought it best to speak his language.

"I hear ya bud. I'm going to say it this way. I believe that the big guy upstairs gave each and every one of us our miraculous bodies and wants us to take care of them, to be the best we can be, no matter what."

Jake agreed. "Hundred per cent!"

I continued. "Now if you knew that at birth you were given a Ferrari, and it was yours to keep and do with as you pleased, would you leave it out in the rain? Put stale gas in it? Never check the oil? Let the tires go flat?"

"Not a chance dude! Great analogy!" he said.

"I think if people realized how precious, how high performance, how valuable our bodies really are, they would take way better care of them. And as far as we really know, we only get one. So I'm taking my Ferrari for regular runs to clean the carbon out. I'm only putting high-test fuel in it and I'm changing the oil in it like clockwork! Mine's gonna be on that track racing right to the very end. No malfunctions due to negligence for me! " I said.

Transferable Life Skill

Even if your car is just "A to B" for you, take darn good care of it. The last thing you want is for it to let you down when you need it most, because you didn't look after it. Look after all of your precious valuables, your health, your family, your career. It doesn't really take much time and it will pay back HUGE dividends.

PART 3

20% Exercise

As a personal trainer, I just had to add this part. I get way too many questions on a daily basis to believe that people know what they're actually doing in the playground (let's get this straight... children can usually stay fit by going to the playground every day. We, as adults don't take the time to play, or to go to the playground. The gym IS our playground, except MY playground. It's the Sacred Chamber)!

This is not an exercise book. It's really more about the mental game you need to understand in order to succeed at exercise. Following are some of the techniques and methods that will get you great results in the playground, and when transferred to other areas of your life, will have a profound effect on everything else you do.

CHAPTER 61

Jeanette's Story (Mind/Body Control)

You know what you gotta do – now do it

As I took Jeannette through her new program, I got her to focus on her range of motion, her form, her breathing and her mind/body connection. That's where it went upside down. She looked at me quizzically and said, "My what connection?"

I explained. "Researchers were testing Olympic athletes. They had them hooked up to monitors with electrodes and asked them to 'visualize' performing their event.

"They were amazed to see that the very same muscle neurons were firing, and the muscle fibers were twitching that would react on the track had they been actually performing their event!

"Right after, when they turned the athletes loose to perform, the muscles said, 'Oh yeah, we just warmed up. We've already done this. Let's go!' They had muscle memory and achieved greater efficiency.

"They then took the concept to the playground. If you can get your mind into the muscle, actually see the extension and the contraction as you perform the exercise, you will fire more neurons and more muscle fibers, and that leads to more and better results."

Transferable Life Skill

Visualization is the key to getting the results you're aiming for. The gift of imagination is what separates us from the rest of the creatures on the planet. As Napoleon Hill said, "Whatever the mind of

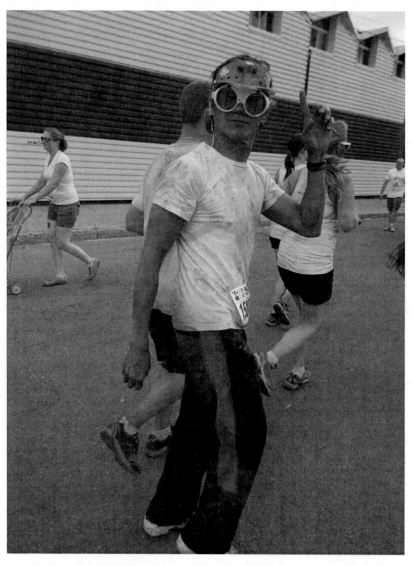

Colour Me Rad Fun Run with windshield wiper sunglasses!
Photo by Amanda Jean Malbeuf

man can conceive and believe, it can achieve." Program your sub-conscious mind with the picture of success in everything you want to do, have or be. It will follow through to completion if you keep focused, keep repeating the message, and act. ALWAYS see a positive outcome! NEVER visualize failure! Your subconscious mind will act on what it sees!

This is the reason that a lot of fitness competitors use pictures of their heroes in the playground to motivate and inspire them. In fact, one of the Body for Life competitors actually put a picture of Frank Zane, a famous bodybuilder, on his fridge, and superimposed a picture of his own head on Frank's so that he could see himself with the body of his dreams.

CHAPTER 62

Cory's Story (Breathing Control)

Success is not an accident

"Man, I just can't get the breathing thing down. I can't get my head around it. Is it really that important?" Cory asked between halted breaths.

As I raised my hands and crossed my index fingers I said, "Here are a couple of tricks to help you. Try to remember the two X's. Whenever you 'eXert' the muscle, that's when you 'eXhale'. Watch this."

I mimicked an arm curl for him. "When my arm is at the bottom of the range of motion I'm not exerting the muscle. This is 'initiation'. ALWAYS take a deep breath here. When I raise the weight to the top of the range of motion, that's where I'm 'eXerting' the muscle so that's when I 'eXhale'. Two X's... and ALWAYS inhale on 'initiation'. These two techniques work with all playground exercises.

"If you breathe in this way, you will always be able to do more reps and lift more weight. That's the name of the game! That's how you get results!

"In fact, Doc Miller's wife, Yanni, told me that she now uses the breathing technique whenever she goes up and down stairs. Lift leg, breathe in, step down, and breathe out. She can do stairs all day long."

Transferable Life Skill

Find neat little ways to remember how to do the fundamentals and then DO them. They will become second nature and you won't have to consciously think about them later. You'll be automatically creating more efficiency.

CHAPTER 63

Sandy's Story (Cardio vs Resistance Training)

Growth – not comfort

It was 1999 and I was at the YMCA looking out the window of the fitness office onto the exercise floor. I watched Sandy spend a half hour on the treadmill, a half hour on the elliptical trainer, and then yet another half hour on the recumbent bike. I approached her. "Sandy, I'm having a 'psychic day' today. I'm getting the feeling that today is 'fat burning day'! Am I right?"

"Darn right," she squeaked between breaths.

"Can I share some information with you about cardio training?" I offered.

"Please do," she puffed.

I continued. "First, if you look at a graph showing your fat burn, the line doesn't soar straight up the minute you hit the machine and continue in that direction until you fall off onto the floor. It's a very gradual uphill curve. Your body needs to 'ramp up' to get into its fat burning zone. It needs to warm up the muscles and the joints, up-regulate stress hormones, and get through a couple of energy systems before it starts to burn fat. So just because you go on three cardio pieces doesn't mean that you'll burn three times as much fat. The body is an incredible survival mechanism. It doesn't want to keep burning fat. It wants to survive. The line on the graph will flatten out. You'll plateau and then the line drops off. There's a point of diminishing returns. Also, you only get a three or four hour after-burn following cardio training. Would you be interested in a 24-hour fat burn where you could burn fat while you're reading, watching TV, or even while you're surfing the net?"

Her eyes got as big as saucers. "Oh yeah! Bring it!"

"Okay then. We need to get you into the resistance area to regain the lean mass that you've lost over the years. Those years when you could virtually eat whatever you wanted and you didn't put on weight. People typically lose about a half pound of muscle per year after the age of 20 if they're not training properly. And muscle is your metabolic engine."

She hesitated. "Uh... lifting weights?"

I had encountered this before. "Sandy, your enthusiasm is underwhelming."

"I... I really don't want to do that!" she stuttered.

"Why not?" I asked, knowing fully what the answer would be.

"I don't want to look like Arnold Schwarzenegger!" she stated.

I looked directly at her. "Sandy, you're never going to look like Arnold for three reasons. One, you don't have enough testosterone in your system to look like Arnold. Boys have 10 times that of girls. Two, you won't be in the playground five to six hours a day like Arnold was in order to get that way. And three, IF for some unknown reason, you're a 'genetic mutant' and you put on gobs and gobs of muscle, I'll take you off the 'transformation' program and put you on a 'maintenance' program. How would that be?"

Still looking horrified, she tried to be nice. "Uh Randy, I... I don't think so."

So I apologized for interrupting her workout. "Ok Sandy, you're our member. You're driving the bus. Sorry for bothering you! Carry on!"

Three years later I was, again, looking out the window of the fitness office onto the exercise floor. I saw Sandy spend a half hour on her treadmill, a half hour on her elliptical trainer, and then finish with her usual half hour on her recumbent bike. This saddened me. I approached her. "Sandy, can I do a 'Doctor Phil' on you?"

"Sure," she panted.

"How's this working for you?"

In obvious despair she said, "Ok, it isn't. What should I do?"

"Well, I see you in here regularly working out, and with your determination, commitment, and perseverance, you deserve results. It's just not fair for you to be that dedicated and not get the outcome you're striving for. If you're not hitting your goals you may as well be doing something else."

"That's for sure, it's depressing."

I took her cue. "Ok, how about we get some results now?"

"Let's do it!" she said with renewed enthusiasm.

That day we started a proper resistance training program. Five months later, Sandy was "strutting" through the gym sporting a gorgeous aqua spandex outfit, lifting gloves, and what I call a "belly shirt". You know... the ones where you can see her abs. And she had abs!

I regularly have women sitting in the office with me as I go over their medical and exercise history. At that time I always ask them for their "specific" goal so that we have something concrete to aim for. I can't tell you how many times a woman has looked out onto the exercise floor, pointed to Sandy, and said to me, "I'd like to look like her!"

At which point I will often say, "Let me tell you a little story about... her!"

Transferable Life Skill

Doing the same thing over and over again, expecting a different result would be the very definition of insanity. Often the most effective way to do a job is to take the proven, more difficult route. Always keep an open mind. In most cases it will save you time. If you do what's easy and comfortable, your life will end up difficult and uncomfortable, but if you do the difficult and uncomfortable, your life will be easier and more comfortable. Never take the easy way out.

CHAPTER 64

Manjit's Story (NWMO)

Don't envy the champion – BE the champion

"I love doing my cardio. I just want to lose more fat with my cardio sessions!" she said adamantly.

I shook my head. "Manjit, in the early 1980's, a gal by the name of Rachel McLish was winning all kinds of body building awards and was Ms. Olympia a number of times. She said, 'Ladies if you think you're going to lose fat by dieting and doing cardio alone, think again. You WILL lose fat but you will also lose water and muscle. So when you walk by the mirror you will simply see a smaller fat person. What you really want to see is all the nice curves, and those curves are muscle!'

"There's a condition we call NWMO, normal weight metabolically obese, or skinny fat. For a guy, this is the person who can walk into a men's store and buy a suit right off the rack, and with a little sleeve and pant hemming he's good to go. But ask this guy to take off his shirt and, 'Houston we have a problem!' He's skinny. He's got no muscle! At best, that lack of muscle also leads to physical dysfunction, lack of energy, lack of strength and endurance, and an overall lack of optimal health, and at worst, a risk of injury.

"Now I'm sure you have friends who everyone thinks looks great because they're thin and they look 'normal' in clothes. But really, when they're in a bathing suit, you could turn them sideways, ask them to stick out their tongue and they'd look like a zipper.

"I'm not saying to forego your cardio sessions. I'm just saying that you need to add resistance training into the mix so that you don't look skeletal."

Almost tearfully she asked, "Can I still do my cardio?"

"Fersure!"

Transferable Life Skill

Don't let appearances fool you. Often what appears to be desirable is not always where you really want to be. Believe it or not, there are actually some people who hide things they don't want others to see. It would be surprising to find out how much they would love to be a better version of themselves. Go the distance. Become the very best YOU can be.

CHAPTER 65

Dani's Story (Cardio Frequency)

If it doesn't challenge you – it won't change you

Dani was a "hard gainer", someone who has to work really hard to put on muscle, and she had to eat like a porker. I think her main problem was that she just loved to run. One day she caught me at the desk. "Do you have any suggestions for me to get more definition?"

"Dani, I see you in here regularly doing two hour long cardio sessions. That's crazy! Are you training for a marathon?"

"No, I just feel good when I run," she answered.

"Well, pardon the pun, but which would make you feel better in the long run? Hitting the treadmill every day or having that great definition you asked about, with something to define?"

"Both," she answered.

"Alright, so you like to have your cake and eat it too, huh?" I said. "First I need to let you know that too much cardio is muscle wasting, exactly opposite of your goal if definition is what you're looking for.

"Have you ever looked closely at long-distance runners or people who do a lot of marathons each year?"

She admitted, "Can't say that I have."

"Ok, no names here but one famous world class marathon runner is 5'9" and a 130 pounds and another is 5'10" and 134 pounds. When they take their shirts off they look emaciated. You actually want to point them in the direction of the nearest buffet!

"My suggestion? I would quit the cardio for a few months and get in the weight room. First, you have to have some muscle to define. And increase your calories by 50 per cent. Then let's take a look-see at the results and decide where we may need to adjust. You'll put on a bit of fat while doing this but don't worry. We can shear off fat way faster and easier than putting on muscle."

Transferable Life Skill

If you continue to do what you always have, you will continue to have what you've always had. Just because you like to do a certain part of the job doesn't mean that it's the most productive way to spend your time. Often, doing what you like to do will not take you to the goal as quickly as doing what you may not enjoy as much. Recognize who and what you are. Then do what needs to be done.

CHAPTER 66

Mike's Story (Cardio Intensity)

Bring on the fire

One day after finishing up a program with a member, I had a few minutes to kill, so I was patrolling the exercise floor looking for people I could torture... uh, help.

Mike waved me over from a recumbent bike. "Can I ask you a question? I'm a little confused here."

"Uh oh, confusion is not good, Mike. How may I be of service?" I asked.

"Some of the trainers are telling me that I should be pedaling fast and others are telling me I should be pedaling slowly. Which is it?"

"Ok, Mike. My turn. Can I ask you two questions?"

"Sure, hit me."

"First, what's your goal?"

"I just want to lose a few pounds of fat around my waist."

I continued. "Ok, second question. Do you know what fuel your body prefers to burn?"

He looked at me quizzically. "What do you mean?"

"Well, your body wants to burn sugar and carbohydrate calories. It doesn't want to burn fat! It's an incredible survival machine. It wants to store fat. That's how humans stayed on the planet.

"The only time that you can burn fat is in an arena of oxygen. Here's an example. In order for this room to catch on fire, we would need three things: fuel to burn, a spark to light it, and oxygen. The same is required in your body: fat to burn, muscle firing to light it, and oxygen. So if I come up to you while you're on this bike and I ask you what you had for brekky and you're pedaling so hard you can't get any words out... you're in an anaerobic state - without oxygen. Every breath you're taking is coming in to keep you alive. There's nothing extra to burn fat. Now on the other hand, let's say that when I ask about your morning menu, you can actually string a couple of sentences together before you need to take a breath. Now you're in an aerobic state - with oxygen... and that provides the extra oxygen to help you burn fat."

"Oh, ok, so I should be pedaling slowly?"

"Yep, you want to do LSD," I joked. "No, not the drug... 'Long-Slow-Distance'. But there's a corollary to the rule. And that is... most people have no problem doing the 'Slow' in LSD... but they don't want to do the 'Long Distance'. It's human nature to want to conserve energy. So if you have 45 minutes to an hour or so, you can go slower to burn fat. But if you only have 20 minutes, I'd suggest doing intervals. Although you won't be burning as many fat calories, you could burn more calories quicker, and at the end of the day, fat loss requires a caloric deficit."

Transferable Life Skill

Learn and study all the different methods to acquire your goal. Don't confuse them. Always use the method that works best for your intention and the goal that you're striving for. Learning and studying are lifelong endeavors in every area of your life. You must never stop. The person who doesn't continue learning is no better than the one who can't.

CHAPTER 67

Bev's Story(The Squat/Giving Up)

Life has its ups and downs – we call them squats

Bev dejectedly announced, "No more squats for me. I think I tweaked my back last week."

Concerned, I looked at her. "How much does it hurt right now? What level of pain are you feeling?"

She admitted, "Well, nothing right now. It was just for a few seconds after my last set."

I got the picture. "So really, the issue is that you don't like doing squats?"

"Yeah, I guess so," she agreed.

"Bev, I'm not telling you that you absolutely have to do squats, but when a survey was done with bodybuilders asking the question, 'If there was only one exercise that you could do for the rest of your life. What would it be?' They unanimously said, 'The squat... because it uses so many muscles!'

"The trick is to do it right! Try to keep an upright position, a straight back. Never lean forward because the heavy weight will cause you to fire the little muscles at the small of your back and that gets ugly. Also keep your toes behind your knees to protect the joints. Now, I know that this is rather controversial in the power lifting circles where they do get their knees way past their toes but here in our playground we always err on the side of safety."

I then showed her my "squatting hand puppet". (You can find it at nowgogetpumped.com)

"However, right now, I would take some time to recover. Or if it's bad, see a physio about your back. But then get back to squats as soon as you can. Squats are the exercise that will keep you from needing help getting off a toilet seat when you're 80 years old. They're most definitely your best friends!"

Transferable Life Skill

Don't give up on the things that count just because you don't like them. Imagine not brushing your teeth because you don't like it.

Typically if you like an exercise, you probably don't need it as much as the one you dislike. Find out how to do all things properly and keep at it. You just may find the challenge to be invigorating, and most certainly worth the effort. You might actually get to like it!

CHAPTER 68

Cal's Story (Order Cardio/ Resistance)

Let's go burn some calories

If I've finished a program with a member and they're good to go, I like to wander around the playground floor and hunt down other members who look like they may need some help. I respond best to screams.

On this particular day, Cal was really working up a nice sweat on an upright bike. "Hey dude," he said as he wiped his forehead. "I read somewhere that it makes a difference whether you do cardio or resistance training first. What's your take?"

"Well," I answered, "as with almost everything, that can be fairly controversial, but I believe, that if you're doing them both on the same day, and if you're working out for the reason that most people do, to burn fat, that you should do cardio at the end of your playground session."

"Because?"

"Resistance training will ramp up your stress hormones and deplete some of your glycogen stores, which will help you get into your fat-burning zone quicker, as opposed to taking more time to get there if you do your cardio training first. That way, as soon as you get onto your cardio equipment, you're burning fat almost immediately."

He frowned. "But I always find that I'm too gassed after a heavy weight session and I struggle to do the cardio if I wait until the end."

"In that case, I would dial the intensity of the cardio back a bit so that you can still finish it. You can always progress it as you do with your other exercises," I offered.

"What would happen if I did the cardio before resistance?"

"First, it would take longer to get into your fat-burning zone. Essentially your entire session would take longer. And second, you may find that you can't lift the same loads if you're training legs."

He pushed further. "It kinda sounds like a no-win situation to me. Got a better idea?"

"I might suggest a split routine would work better for you. Resistance one day, cardio the next day, repeat. That way, you could max out both systems on different days."

"Now, THAT sounds like a plan!" he said with a huge grin. "I could do that."

Transferable Life Skill

There are always methods to "hack" a situation to find the most efficient way to get the job done. Educate yourself to find the options, then get creative, experiment and find what works best for you, given your time limits, preferences, and goals.

CHAPTER 69

Larry's Story(Exercise Order)
For things to change – you gotta change

"Hey, great to see you Larry. How's your program going?" I asked one of our newest members who was just getting used to his brand new program.

He replied, "I came in and did my upper body program yesterday. It was pretty busy and I couldn't get the equipment I wanted, so I was a little out of order with my exercises. That's ok, right?"

"Give me an example," I said.

"I couldn't get a bench for my dumbbell chest press. They were all being used. But I found a tricep pull down so I did that first, until I could get a bench."

I shook my head. "Oooopsies, Lar. Not the best idea. The smaller muscles are very often the secondary movers for the larger primary muscles. For instance, in your bench press, the pecs are your primary movers, the triceps are the secondaries. So if you're wandering around the playground and you can't get a bench because they're all being used, don't head on over and work your triceps. You depend on them for the press and if you pre-fatigue them before you do your chest press, you'll be wondering why you can't get a maximum lift for your pecs! You're not gonna be a happy camper when those weights knock your teeth onto the floor!"

"Yeah, I couldn't figure out why I was having such a problem lifting the same weight as I did last time. I thought I was just having a bad day," he admitted.

I quickly followed up. "Same thing when training your back. Don't gas your biceps before working your back. You won't get a maximum lift because you'll have pooched those secondaries, and that will blow your 'personal best' for that muscle group as well.

"I'll always strategically set up your program to reflect the most efficient training patterns, larger muscles to smaller muscles. Best not to train them out of order," I said.

Transferable Life Skill

Don't go into anything "willy nilly". Have a logical well thought out plan and do things in the order that creates the greatest result. Some things depend on factors that are not always apparent. Learn true efficiency and use those methods.

CHAPTER 70

AJ's Story (Progression)
You don't deserve it – you earn it

"No matter what I do, I just can't increase the weight on this exercise," AJ said, stating an often repeated lament heard throughout the playground.

I felt his pain. "Otay... it *has* been quite a few weeks, and you've been progressing the weight regularly so genetically you could be close to your max. But try this little trick, and beat your genetics. If the set requires say, 12 reps, your goal now is 13 reps. Once you can get the 13 reps, the next goal is 14 reps. Once you can do 14 reps, drop the reps back down to 12 but increase the weight five pounds. You might not be able to get 12 reps with the new weight, maybe only 10 or 11, but shoot for the 12. Once you can get the 12, repeat that procedure a couple of times. Then we'll change the exercise. You've just experienced 'the Ceiling Principle and Micro Progression!'"

AJ spent another two weeks on his program and was able to increase his weight by 20 per cent.

Transferable Life Skill

Don't be surprised when the huge progress at the start of a program slows down and it feels like it's taking forever to reach the goal. Stay the course. You can break through any plateau in any undertaking. Sometimes you just need to "challenge" yourself in different ways.

CHAPTER 71

Kylie's Story (Travelling)
Rituals define you

"I'm heading to Hawaii next week. What do you do for exercise when you're on holidays or travelling?" Kylie asked.

"First Kylie, let me say this. I'll carry your luggage for you if you get me an airplane ticket," I offered.

By the look on her face I could tell that wasn't going to happen.

So I got all serious. "In the past we would always book a hotel with a playground. It was a deal breaker! No playground, no reservation.

"If our destination didn't have hotels with playgrounds, at the very least we would do sets of multi-joint, compound body-weight exercises. However, a number of years ago our supervisor emailed me and asked if I would be interested in taking a TRX course. I told him, 'I'm ALWAYS interested in learning anything new. I'm your man!'

"Because I had been training people since way back in 1974, I have a pretty refined 'crap o meter'! I've seen all kinds of fad diets and fad equipment come and go. I've seen the vibro belts, the ab toners, the thigh busters, the ab loungers, the shake weights, the fit flops, the power bracelets... all kinds of late-night buck grabbers.

"But when I took the TRX course, my meter didn't even peep once.

"TRX was developed by Navy Seals. When they were on a mission in the field of war, they didn't have any equipment or playgrounds to maintain their physical skills. So they would take their karate belts and hang them over tree branches, in doorways, or the gun barrels on the turrets of the tanks and do suspension training. ABSolutely brilliant!

"The motto for TRX is 'All Core, All the Time' and it works.

"We take our TRX wherever we travel… to Mexico, Hawaii, even Vegas, where they have these exorbitant, totally ridiculous 'resort fees' to use their playgrounds. We'll just hook up to a closet door and we're in business.

"Or we'll be on the beach before anybody gets up. The sun is rising, the surf is coming in and we have our TRX hooked up to a palapa. ABSolutely gorgeous! We finish our workout and head in for a nice brekky buffet to repair tissue and ramp up our glycogen stores!"

Kylie looked a little sheepish and said, "But what if I can't afford a TRX? It took all my cash to pay for the trip."

"No worries. Body-weight exercises are your friends. Find a tree or a cross beam somewhere and do pull ups. Push-ups, dips, squats, lunges, calf raises and bicycle crunch twists will hit all the major muscle groups. All of these will keep you from deconditioning until you get home. Add swimming, surfing, beach running, snorkeling, and sail boarding and you'll come back in better shape than when you left. You'll be a hurtin unit!

"Heck, if you twist my arm, I'll give you my world famous Killer Abs program. My wife and I have had fellow hotel patrons doing them on the beach with us in Mexico. C'mon I'll show you!"

We only did 10 reps and Kylie was crying like a little baby.

Between breaths she said, "Geez man, when you said, 'let's do 10' I thought it was going to be easy."

Laughing, I looked at her. "Well, it WAS 10… 10 of each movement, 15 movements all together. Congrats. You just did 150 reps total! Gee… that's a 150 more reps than most people do in their entire lives! And no sniveling, we do 100 reps of each movement, 1500 in total, for our Strong Kids Campaign Fund Raiser for the YMCA."

"They should lock you up dude!" she said with a total lack of respect.

"Hey, don't make me come over there and violate my parole," I joked. "I'll lay a Bumpa Beating on ya! That's Killer Abs I… when you can do 50, you get to do Killer Abs II (the Sequel)… then, when you can do 50 of those, you earn the right to do Killer Abs III (Son of Killer Abs)!"

"Anybody ever get to Killer Abs II?" she asked with a look of sheer horror on her face.

"Only two people… and they quit after trying it a couple of times because the first exercise is V-ups. They went back to Killer Abs I."

"Anybody get to three?" she gulped.

"Nope!"

Transferable Life Skill

There is more than one way to get the job done. Don't allow excuses to stop you from maintaining your healthy lifestyle. Always plan. It can be difficult to get back into your routine after a layoff. Many times you will need to improvise to achieve the goal. There are lots of cool creative ways to get results. Remember, don't be upset by the results you didn't get from the workout you didn't do!

Be brave. Give it a go. Try the infamous Killer Abs Program at now-gogetpumped.com

CHAPTER 72

Carly's Story (Bodybuilding)
Redefine yourself

I was introduced as a super-fun personal trainer to Carly at a seminar and I could tell what she was going to say by the way she looked me up and down at our first meeting. "Can I ask you a personal question?"

"Shoot!"

"Why don't you look like a trainer?" she asked.

"You mean, why don't I look like a bodybuilder?"

"Yeah!"

"Well, my personal belief is that bodybuilding is pretty extreme. It's very hard on a person, the training, the diet, the dehydration, and the sacrifices. Clothes have to be custom made to look good, and then after all that, the results only last for a few days. I'm more interested in functional training. I train 'go muscles', not 'show muscles'."

"But don't you care what people think when they meet you and they learn that you're a trainer?" she asked.

"If people think that I have to be a bodybuilder to be a great trainer, they need to give their toques a spin. Now, I'm not saying that a personal fitness trainer shouldn't be fit. Having an obese personal trainer would be kinda like having a suicidal life coach. I'm just saying that he doesn't need to be a bodybuilder.

"Allow me to tell you a story. A few years ago I was talking to another drummer buddy of mine and I asked him, 'Frank, why is it that we don't see more drummers with touring bands, playing electronic drums on stage?'

"He just scowled and said, 'Coz, they're ugly!'

"Look, I know your drum instructor uses electronic drums. Ask him for me will ya?" I said, ignoring the dirty look.

"The next time I saw Frank, I asked, 'So what did your drum teacher tell you?'

"He informed me that his drum teacher told him that electronic drums are easier to tear down and set up, they never go out of tune, they always have the same stick response, and they can give you over 400 different sounds and dozens of custom kit sounds at a twist of a dial.

"When Frank interjected with, 'but they're ugly', his drum instructor's response was (as the folks at MasterCard once said, 'priceless'), 'Frank, I'm sixty-two years old, I don't give a rat's patootie what anybody thinks!'"

Turning to Carly I said, "So that's exactly the way I feel about what people think of me! I train for function and strength. I maintain my body fat below 11 per cent and now that I'm in my sixties, I really don't give a rodent's butt what anybody thinks!"

Transferable Life Skill

Feel comfortable in your own skin. Don't let others dictate the way you think. Your self-image is more important than what anyone else may think of you.

Dr. Steven Covey has a book called *Primary Greatness*. It's about character, honor, perseverance, integrity, service, self-sacrifice and contribution!

"Secondary Greatness" is all about impressions, position, image… how big is the house, what kind of car, and are they designer clothes? Who cares? Answer - nobody worthwhile! Don't become a "label victim"!

Some people spend money they don't have on things they don't need to impress people they don't even like!

CHAPTER 73

Ann's Story (Machines vs Free Weights)
Good things come to those who sweat

Ann was 37 years old and she was a newbie in the training department. She was a little apprehensive. "I don't mind telling you, this is a little scary for me. I've never been in a gym before. All this equipment, it's really daunting. People will laugh at me. I'm afraid I'll look like an idiot. What can I do so I don't attract attention?"

I tried to ease her fear. "No worries. I look like an idiot all the time.

"When I get someone who has never played with weights or experienced our playground, I usually set up their first program on machines. They're safer than free weights and can be adjusted for your personal range of motion. They'll develop muscle memory and don't require as much technique!

"However, I want to get you off the machines as soon as possible because you'll get way more results from free weights. Machines isolate the muscles that you're using and don't fire the stabilizers like free weights do."

As I expected, she looked at me quizzically and shrugged her shoulders. "So should we start with that contraption?" she asked, pointing toward a Smith machine.

"Actually, that's more of a hybrid, a good transition, between machines and free weights. It's great if you don't have a spotter.

"Here, let me explain a little further. If you're doing a chest press on a machine, you push the bars in one direction and you usually don't have the luxury of any other directional movements. However, when you use a barbell (the long bar), lie on your back and perform that exact same movement, you have to balance the bar to keep it from wobbling all over the place. That takes more stabilizer muscles to balance it.

"Now, if you really want a lot of muscle recruitment, use dumbbells (the short bars). Again, on that same movement, one arm is wobbling around wanting to come down and rip your arm off and the other wants to come crashing down on your skull! Gee mom, look at all those stabilizers at work. The more muscle you recruit, the more results you get."

"Ok, I guess it's machines for the first program then."

I smiled. "Ann, I'm going to set up each machine for your individual body type and the length of your levers, and I'll write the settings down on your exercise card so you don't have to guess every time you come into the playground. You'll look like a pro!"

Transferable Life Skill

How do you eat an elephant? One bite at a time! Don't bite off more than you can chew. You'll get sick. Take little bites, and eventually the whole elephant is gone! Wow! Look what you did! See the big picture and progress bits at a time.

CHAPTER 74

Allan's Story (Core stability)
Success is an inside/out process

"What are you doing for core training?" I asked, after Allan told me that his mom, a long-time client, wanted me to train him for his hockey season.

He shrugged his shoulders. "Nothing. Our coach only has us doing drills. You know, skating, stick handling, passing, shooting... that stuff."

I was shocked. "Allan, that 'stuff' is really important but let me get all 'Asian' on you here! Asian people will tell you that ALL of your power comes from your center. Your core is your center. A strong core provides the stability for the extremities to drive off of. A strong core equals more power and control. If we strengthen your core, you will be able to accelerate faster, change directions quicker and stop on a dime and give change! Interested?"

"You bet!" he replied with enthusiasm. "My mom has one of those 'ball in a cradle chairs'. I'll start using it."

"Not so quick dude. The cradle defeats the purpose of sitting on the ball. It creates stability which is opposite of the effect you're looking for. Sit on a regular ball for better results," I cautioned.

After a few months of core training with a real stability ball, wobble boards and Bosus, Allan had his best hockey season... ever!

Transferable Life Skill

Sometimes what appears to be unrelated is the basic key to achieving the goal. Think about the benefits of doing something seemingly unrelated and you may be pleasantly surprised to see how it can accelerate your success in the big picture.

CHAPTER 75

TheKim's Story (The Kick-up)
Do it with authority

Please don't think that I'm "dissing" my wife!!! I call her "TheKim" because of a Yul Brynner movie, "The King and I". Hence, "TheKim&I".

For almost 40 years, TheKim had never stepped into a playground! Pretty sad. Then she met me! Uh oh!

She read me the riot act right away. "If you become an alcoholic, I'm leaving you!" She obviously had an interesting past.

I replied with my priority. "If you become obese, I'M leaving YOU!"

So far, so good! Neither of us has come close to the door.

TheKim gets up every morning and hits the playground with me at five am. She does the same routine that I do and she's VERY strong and VERY functional! You want this girl on your team in any competition.

Now, having said that, there was a time when she was having difficulty getting her dumbbell chest press up to a decent weight.

"In order to progress and get better results, you have to get past this plateau," I said. "You should be able to lift more weight."

"How? I can't even get the heavier weights into position," she said, almost dropping them onto the playground floor.

"Try the kick-up with momentum. Use your legs to drive the heavier weights into position."

"Explain," she demanded.

"Sit on the end of the bench," I said. "Find the sweet spot at 90 degrees. Put the weights on the very end of your knees to get the right leverage. Now stand up. And as you sit down throw your knees up quickly, using momentum, drive the weights up to the ceiling, keeping your arms straight.

"In your mind, think 'slam these things right into the ceiling' with your legs and your arms! Imagine a giant electro-magnet pulling the weights to the ceiling!" I said, as I demonstrated for her with two 90 pound dumbbells.

"You'll be able to lift crazy weights, and that'll allow you to progress and start getting results again!

"Now let's make sure that you can complete the movement, so that you don't injure your rotator cuffs by dropping the weights on the floor by your side. Once you finish your set, bring your knees up. 'Hammer' your knees with the weights. Lock your hips and the weights will fire you into a standing position. This technique is super-efficient. The trick will be to not shoot yourself across the playground into a mirror when you stand up... unless you're wearing your helmet, of course."

TheKim can now lift 45 pound dumbbells, not bad for a tiny 5'3", 66 year old fire cracker! She won't turn green but you still don't ever want to see her angry!

Transferable Life Skill

Stop when you stall out at anything. Look at what you can do to make the process easier or more efficient, and adapt. Often, there will be a useful technique that you need to incorporate to get the job done more efficiently. For a video demo of the "kick-up", go to nowgogetpumped.com

CHAPTER 76

Gio's Story(Perfect Form)

Growing old is mandatory – growing up is optional

Gio was kidding around with a friend in the playground when he turned to me and let me in on their conversation. "Winter's coming and we're wondering what might be a great exercise to help us prevent falling on the ice and snow this year."

Even though Gio and his bud are chronologically enhanced (both 76 years young), I suggested, "Howzbout a nice Bosu body-weight squat? That'll fire the ol' core and ramp up your balance and co-ordination."

Gio frowned. "We might be a bit old to be using those Bosu things."

I assured them both. "Old? You're both just pups. You're not even close to your 'best-before dates'."

Now just because they're both seniors, doesn't mean that they're not adventurous. "Let's do this!" they chorused.

After I grabbed a couple of Bosus and demonstrated the exercise for them, they eagerly jumped on and gave it the ol' college try. They were doing quite well when one of the other trainers came over and asked to yak with me privately.

"They don't have perfect form and their ranges of motion suck," she said to me.

I was somewhat ticked off that this trainer would interrupt a session to provide her opinion, but I was my usual nicey nice about the situation so I just said, "They both have compromised knee joints from years of extreme activities. So that's why I've only programmed a partial range of motion. Also, I know that they're slightly leaning forward, but they aren't using any weights at all, and they're definitely safe. It's their first set, ever. And neither of them is in a bodybuilding contest, so isolation is not the priority and just because they're using a few more muscles to help them get the job done, it isn't necessarily a bad thing."

I actually wanted to say MYOB... but that's not my style (in public).

We turned to look at Gio and his friend. They were playing on the Bosu and having more fun than a barrel of people!

Transferable Life Skill

Perfectionism can be debilitating. As long as you're safe, get the job done with as much help from your survival friends as you can. The last person who was perfect had nail holes in his hands.

CHAPTER 77

Jennifer's Story(Modality)
You can die in the bleachers or you can die in the field

"I'm not so sure that I'm getting into this resistance thing. I mean, the dumbbells and all," Jennifer notified me as she sat up from a rather wobbly inclined dumbbell fly.

"What? Please tell me you're having as much fun as I am!" I said.

"You should come to my Pilates class with me and see how hard I work out," she said.

"Let's not and say we did," I demanded.

"What's your take on Pilates?" she responded with an obvious ulterior motive.

"Whoa, this is a trick question, right? Is anybody recording our conversation?" I asked, looking around the playground for a bug.

"Oh, c'mon," she demanded. "What's your opinion? Really! You never say anything when I tell you about my Pilates classes."

Keeping my voice down I said, "Ok, Jennifer, just between us girls, I've taken a number of Pilates courses at our Fitness Instructor's Spring and Fall Training Retreats and I have to say, that every single time, I'm always left wondering what we're going to do for exercise right after the session. I just don't feel that I've had a work out! I want to go for a run or do some pull ups... something, anything!

"Jennifer, I believe that Pilates is great for sofa spuds who have never exercised a day in their lives and are just starting their fitness journey... or perhaps someone recovering from an accident. But your goal is transformation, and done properly, there is NOTHING that will change your body as much as free weights! " I added. "You asked for my opinion!"

Has there ever been a time in your life when you just knew that you said something that was going to come back and bite you in the butt later? This, was one of those times. Ouch!

When I saw Jennifer for her next playground session she put me on notice. "I told my Pilates instructor what you said about Pilates."

"Oh perfect. Just what the doctor ordered," I thought to myself.

Jennifer continued. "She said that you have an open invitation to go to her studio any time and she'll put you through a Pilates program that will change your tune."

I was somewhat shocked that she played the recording to her instructor. "Ok, tell her no problem. I whole-heartedly accept her challenge. She can give me the whole meal deal. But only under one condition: that she comes to my playground right after so that I can return the favor and put her through one of my programs. Then I promise I'll call the ambulance to take her to the hospital!"

Oddly, I never did hear from her instructor!

Transferable Life Skill

As Jack Reacher once said in one of his movies when he was challenged to a fight by four punks - "Remember, you asked for this!" It's never a wise move to make challenges unless you're absolutely positive you're going to win. And even then, remember, there's always someone better, faster, or stronger! How did the great thinker put it? "It's always better to remain quiet and be thought a fool, than to open your mouth and remove all doubt!"

CHAPTER 78

Rob's Story(Intensity)
Start strong – finish stronger

"Wow that was a tough set!" Rob said as he racked the bar.

"Really? You should notify your face. You looked pretty darned relaxed on that final rep," I countered.

"No really, it wasn't easy," he said half convincingly.

"Ok, let's yak about intensity levels," I suggested. "Level one is Rob lying in bed, 'thinking' about getting up. Not too intense right?" He nodded.

"Level 10 would be me taking my flame thrower out of my back pocket and lighting your track pants on fire, and I'm watching you bolting across the parking lot screaming blue murder at the top of your lungs. That's high intensity!"

I continued. "Now level five would be Rob taking two bags of groceries out of the trunk of his car, walking them into the house and putting them onto the kitchen table. Most people tell me that's not very intense. But I would say, why don't you sit your bum down in that kitchen chair beside those groceries? You may find that your heart is beating faster, your breathing is slightly elevated and perhaps your forehead is not dripping like a dog, but it's slightly moist. That would be a nice 'warm up set', a decent level five."

"But I don't want to start shaking during the level 10 set," he said.

Correction required. "Actually, you do. It's called 'neural activation'. Your body is trying to create new neural pathways so that it can survive the challenge. It's an adaptation response, a survival mechanism. Don't worry about what other people think when they see you shaking. They should be jealous! For effective transformation, your goal and their goal should be to get a level 10 intensity on the final rep of the last set for each muscle group!"

"Wow, that's pretty intense!" he said half joking.

I agreed. "Yep, now keep in mind that there will be some days when you can tackle tigers. And other days you'll have your hands clasped together and praying that you can be taken now. The weight is not necessarily the goal. It's intensity!"

Transferable Life Skill

Never push yourself to the point of danger but always challenge yourself to push the envelope. Discomfort creates growth. Earl Nightingale once said, "Most people tip toe through life, hoping they make it safely to death!"

CHAPTER 79

Janet's Story(Self Consciousness)

I am my own hero

Sitting in our office, just before stepping out in to the playground, Janet confessed, "I'm always so embarrassed when I go into the weight area of the gym."

"What exactly are you concerned about, Jan?" I asked.

"Well first, I don't know what I'm doing. And then I'm worried people are looking at me and laughing."

I cautioned her. "I'm going to get a little sexist here, but... a lot of gals feel that way when they first enter the playground. Let me say this about that. Most true gym rats are so focused on their own workouts that they aren't even watching you. And if they aren't focused on their own workout, they should be, coz that would be a huge reason why they aren't getting the results they're looking for.

"Also, if you walked into the playground and saw a big buff guy struggling to do his arm curls with 10 pound dumbbells, what would you think?"

She smiled. "I guess I would think he's a wimp."

"Here's what I think. Perhaps he's recovering from some kind of injury and needs to progress slowly. Or it could be possible that he's already done eight progressive sets peaking at 60 pounds and he's on the bottom of the second half of a heavy pyramid set."

Jan nailed it. "I gotcha. Never judge because I could be wrong."

"Right, and anyone who judges *you*, could be wrong! Fuhgetaboutit!"

Transferable Life Skill

Focus on the important things that need to be done. Don't judge others when you don't know their whole story. They're most likely not paying much attention to you anyway. Get over yourself!

CHAPTER 80

Holly's Story(Grip Strength)
You've done harder things than this

Three quarters of the way through a beautiful dumbbell squat, Holly shrieked, "I CAN'T HANG ON!" as she lost form and prepared to drop the weights.

"It's ok! Put 'em on the bench!" I instructed.

"They're too heavy!" she cried as she hurled them onto the bench.

I assured her. "Actually Holly, you're capable of handling considerably more weight than 35 pounds. All of my female clients and members work their way up to at least 50 pounds so they can max out the average hotel playground. You only have 15 more pounds to go for bragging rights. You're doing really well!"

"TWO 50's? That's 100 pounds! How is that going to happen if I can't hang on to the weights?" she said.

"Wow... you're math is way better than mine," I laughed.

"That's a fact!"

"Look, I hear that all the time just before people give up. But let me tell you, if you just hang in there, pun intended, you'll be rewarded handsomely with increased grip strength AND the FUNtabulous results that come with being able to move more tonnage. Just as with all your training, your muscles will condition, forearms and grip strength included.

"Tell you what, I'll bring my fat grips along to our next playground session," I offered.

She hesitated. "Oh, that doesn't sound good."

I quipped, "Yikes, your enthusiasm is underwhelming."

"What are fat grips?" she stuttered.

"They're portable rubber sleeves that fit over the handles of dumb-bells or a barbell to increase the diameter, which makes it more challenging to hang on to, thereby training and conditioning your grip. You're gonna love 'em!" I assured her.

"Well, I do feel soreness in my forearms after I golf or play tennis so I guess I should increase my grip strength. I just want to be able to golf and play tennis until I'm too old to lace up a pair of court shoes."

To Holly's credit, she stuck with it and can easily hang on to her 50 pound dumbbells while doing her squats, lunges, dead lifts and calf raises.

Transferable Life Skill

When anything seems tough, don't quit. Sometimes, while preparing, training or rehearsing, you have to make things even tougher to make the impossible seem easy. And it will. It's called adaptation and conditioning.

CHAPTER 81

Halley's Story(Warm up)

Make it a great day

Halley had just walked into the playground for her session and greeted me with a question. "We've been training now for over five years and I've always meant to ask you why you never get me to warm up?"

"Whatchoo talkin bout? I ALWAYS get you to warm up!" I said.

"No you don't. You never have me walk or run before our sessions, or even do arm swings or stretches. Isn't that dangerous?" she fired back.

Defence time. "I believe that the very best warm up for any exercise, is the exercise itself, with lower weights and higher reps. That way you can increase your heart rate, prep the specific muscles to be used, and flood synovial fluid into the specific joints and prepare the exact systems that you're going to be training, as opposed to say, jogging around the track prepping your lower body before doing an upper body work out."

"Ok, I guess that's why I've never really been injured while working out," she admitted.

"That's probably true!" I agreed.

Transferable Life Skill

There are plenty of ways to prepare for any situation. Try to be as specific as possible in order to address the exact conditions you're going to face. This is one of the reasons why role playing is so beneficial in so many situations, in business, in relationships, in life.

CHAPTER 82

Joan's Story(Periodization)
Dissatisfaction is a creative state

"Well, here I am!" Joan announced as she walked into the office for her first upgrade. "That last program really worked well. I was pretty surprised. I've never been able to hit over a 120 yards on the golf course before and lately I can hit 175. When I did it the first time I thought it was a wonderful fluke, but now I can do it fairly consistently. It's great!"

I grinned. "FUNtabulous! You can thank me later. Just wait until you see what's next."

"What else is there?" she asked.

"Remember when we first got together? I asked you for your goals and you told me you just wanted to be the very best you could be regarding your health and fitness," I said. "And because your golf season was so important to you at that moment in time, we set up a nice Functional Training Program for you, and it sounds like we were pretty successful."

"That's for sure," she agreed.

"In order to be the very best you can be, I want to periodize your program the same way I do my own," I added.

"Uh oh, this sounds dangerous," she said.

"Yep, it is! I'll call the ambulance. By this time next year, you'll be hitting 220!" I assured her.

"What's the plan?" she asked.

"Ok, here's how I set up my own programs. I do four three month stages. At the beginning of the year right after all the holiday festivities most people will usually be carrying a few extra pounds of yellow goose-like fat. So we do a nice 'Transformation Program' to shear off the Yule-time cookies. For the next stage, I want you to be able to do anything physically that you want with no worries of injury or of being incapable. So that means we do a nice 'Functional Training Program' similar to the one you just completed. Next up, a nice little 'Core Program' coz we Canadians know what's coming down the road. Winter! I don't ever want to hear that you fell on the ice or slipped in the snow. That could mean that you lacked core strength, and that would cause me to pay you a visit and maybe even violate my parole. Right after that we can go into 'Maintenance' until after the holidays and repeat."

"I love it! Let's get started!" she beamed.

Transferable Life Skill

It's often a wise idea to break up your progress in any endeavor into specific stages that address certain aspects of the overall plan. Rather than addressing a lot of components at the same time, it can make the entire project more effective and in most cases more enjoyable.

CHAPTER 83

Skip's Story(Knee Replacement/The Hack)

Your body is the engine – your mind is the engineer

As I passed by Skip in the stretching area, he waved me over and said, "I went to my doc the other day with my aching knee and she said that I should expect my knees to wear out as I get older, that they didn't last forever. She thinks I'll probably need a knee replacement."

I said, "Yikes man, it might be time to change docs! I know lots of people who are on their first pair of knees, even runners, myself included. You seem to be moving pretty good to me, are you feeling any pain?"

"Not right now, but lately I get a little pain while going up my basement stairs," he moaned.

"Skip, I gotta tell you a little story. A few months ago I was in my home playground. I was wearing my weighted vest and I had a couple of pretty heavy weights in my hands. I backed up and cut my foot on the leg of one of the machines. There was blood all over the floor.

"I'm not sure if I ever told you this before but I hate the sight of blood, especially mine!"

"What are you doing? You don't wear shoes in the gym?" he asked.

"Skip, it's a 'playground', not a gym. And the reason we play barefoot is because my wife was wearing orthotics and I told her that she needed to strengthen the muscles in her feet rather than addressing the symptom."

"Is that a wise idea?"

"I may be wrong but I doubt it. If you put a neck brace on right now and wore it for a few months, when you removed it, the muscles would have atrophied and you wouldn't be able to hold your head up. Better to find out why you think you need a neck brace in the first place and handle it."

"Ok, I'll buy that."

"Always address the cause, not the symptom. Anyhoo, I found that I was protecting the foot injury by chronically pronating my foot to keep the weight off of the sore part. I think that caused my MCL to stretch a bit and become inflamed, cos a couple of weeks later I noticed knee pain going up stairs. It kinda freaked me out. I told myself that I was NOT going to get a knee replacement."

He pointed a finger at me. "You're gonna put the knee docs outta business."

"Here's the thing. I was at a party a few years ago. I was having a nice little shop talk with a physician. After about a half hour I said, 'George, what kind of medicine do you practice?' and he said, 'I'm a knee surgeon!'"

"I told him that I had a few clients and members with knee issues and I was trying to help them stabilize and support the knee by strengthening the quads, hamstrings and calves.

"He looked at me, smiled, and said, 'That's exactly what you need to do. Fully 80 percent of the people who come to my clinic for knee replacements don't need them. If they would just do what you're telling them to do they would be fine.'"

"Do you think I should try that?" Skip asked.

"Just let me say that after my accident, I not only protected my foot by compensating with the pronation, but I stopped working my lower body as well to allow healing to take place. That was a mistake.

"I decided that if I wanted to relieve the knee pain, I was going to have to get back on the weights and strengthen those muscles again. After a couple of weeks of progression, I was right back to where I was pre-accident, and the pain totally disappeared. I'm back to a 100 per cent again."

"Ok, I'm definitely doing this," he said with conviction.

Transferable Life Skill

First, don't necessarily buy the first opinion, no matter who gives it to you. Second, analyze the situation diligently and always correct the initial cause of the problem. If you continue to try to relieve the symptom, it will always be there. Third, you can hack most problems by thinking the entire process through and getting creative.

CHAPTER 84

Ray's Story(Counting/ Speeding)

We live for the pump

"Eleventeen... twelveteen... oooopsies... I lost count! Sorry. Anybody counting?" I asked Ray as he continued his alternating bicep curl.

He grunted. "Geez man... it's 10! You're the worst counter ever!"

"Ray, when it comes to counting, there are only three kinds of people... those who can... and those who can't!"

"Did you just hear yourself?" he laughed. "Did you even go to school?"

"Yep, grade three was the hardest four years of my life!" I said. "I told ya not to let me count. You're always gonna get a 'bonus round' if I count! And by the way, gimme your radar detector. You're speeding. With all that momentum, those arms just about want to go all by themselves."

"What's the big deal about speed? I'm just trying to get the job done," he blurted.

"Well first, there's an exercise principle called 'time under tension'. You want to keep the blood in the muscle and get a nice pump. Also, because we're working on hypertrophy, we want to recruit those fast-twitch muscles instead of the slow-twitch endurance muscles. Plus, the more momentum you use, the more sympathetic muscle you use and the greater the chance of injury."

"I haven't been injured yet," he said.

I replied, "And we don't want any injuries either. But you said after the last bi/tri session that we did, that your shoulders were feeling it the next day. DOMS can be very rewarding, but ONLY in the muscles we trained."

"What's DOMS?"

"Delayed onset muscle soreness," I explained. "We didn't do shoulders that day. So I needed to watch your form and range of motion this time, and I noticed that you're initiating the curl with your traps. Just let your arms hang naturally, lock the shoulder, no rotation, and only bend at the elbow. Ok I bought tickets to the gun show. Let the show begin!"

Transferable Life Skill

Even if you have a great team, never assume that everything will go as planned. It's always a good idea to keep a close eye on the whole picture. Also, better to do the job right once the first time than have to go back and do it over again.

CHAPTER 85

Stuart's Story(Symmetry)

Change begins with you

"Whoa! Whoa!" I cautioned Stuart as I witnessed his set of one arm 'creature purls'.

"What?" he asked visibly alarmed.

"Geez Stu, how many reps did I just see you do?" I asked.

"I did ten with my right arm and seven with my left arm. Why?" he said.

"There! I wasn't hallucinating! That's what I thought I saw," I said.

"What's wrong with that? I'm right handed, so I never get as many reps with my left side."

"We should be working towards symmetry," I replied. "If you don't create balance, you have a recipe for injury."

"How so?"

I explained by way of example. "Let's say you've got a fully-loaded wheelbarrow and you're trying to get it from one end of your long driveway to the other. Your chances of dumping that wheelbarrow onto its left side are going to be considerably more likely as your grip strength and bicep on your left side become exhausted. This is the reason we train each side with the same amount of weight for the same number of reps."

He countered. "But what if I can lift more and do more reps with my right?"

"Only do the same weight and reps on your dominant side that you can do with your non-dominant side. But keep progressing the non-dominant side until it catches up. Believe me, balanced muscles are your friends."

"Well, it sorta makes sense," he said.

"Also, along with balancing both sides of your body, always make sure that you train opposing muscle groups to prevent injury as well," I added.

"What do you mean now?" he sighed.

"Don't just train your chest and not your back... your quads and not your hamstrings... your biceps and not your triceps. It's the Principle of Symmetry," I answered.

"Ok, I got it!"

Transferable Life Skill

In most cases in life, balance is very important. Think ego/empathy, flexibility/rigidity, coaching/learning, leading/following, and the big one... work/family. Neglecting one for the other often leads to huge challenges that can be very difficult to recover from at worst, to playing catch up, at best.

CHAPTER 86

Art's Story(Relativity)

Too bad ignorance isn't painful

"Great job on those pull ups Art!" I smiled approvingly. "I just caught the last couple as I came around the corner. How many did you get?"

"Only eight. But I could have done more if you weren't sneaking up on me during my set. I'm not sure I want to keep doing this exercise."

I raised my eyebrow. "You're kidding me, right? Pull ups are the all-time best exercise for your back and you're doing them beautifully. Gorgeous progressions. FUNtabulous range of motion and Pamfastic form. Whatchoo thinkin?"

"You know Big Len?" he asked.

"Sure."

He continued. "Well he was watching me doing my pull ups from across the floor and when I finished he basically dissed me right in front of everyone."

"Yikes! What did he say?"

"He said the only reason I can do pull ups is because I'm a light weight. And he can't because he's heavier," Art added.

"Does that make any sense at all?" I laughed. "Listen. No matter how much you weigh, you should have enough muscle strength to carry your own body weight.

"The Big Guy upstairs blessed us all with a skeletal system and a muscle system to support it. If the two systems are mismatched it's your fault. Sure, Len's got a bigger body, but he's also got bigger muscles. If he can't do pull ups, I'd say he needs to train better or lose some freakin' weight to match his strength. Sheeeesh! I'll go over and Bumpa slap him into next Tuesday."

Art smiled. "Is that what I should say to him next time he talks to me?"

"Art, there's only one corner of the Universe that you can change. That's you. You can't force anyone else to change. They're on their own journey. They have to want to change. The best you can do is motivate or inspire them to change, but ultimately it's their choice."

Transferable Life Skill

Invoke the Law of Relativity. Everything is relative. Is the apple sweet or is it sour? It is neither. Compared to sugar, it could be sour. But compared to a lemon, it's probably sweet. Study all situations fully before passing judgement and don't play the "Yeah but, game". Take responsibility and get the job done.

Remember, don't waste your time trying to force others to change. You don't know their journey. You don't know what they're here to learn. Look after your journey. Learn as much as you possibly can about you.

CHAPTER 87

Mikki's Story(Boooring)
Lack of discipline erodes your psyche

Rolling her eyes, Mikki said, "This weight training stuff is so booor-ing!"

"Wow!" I replied. "Now that's interesting. Most people tell me that cardio is boring, which is probably the reason that they're all watching tvs or reading while they're doing it. I never hear that from people doing their resistance training... correctly."

"What do you mean, correctly?"

"Mikki, you drive a car, yes?"

"Of course."

"When you're driving down the street, you need to be focused on your speed, traffic ahead and all around you, signs and signals, how your car is performing, emergency indications, road conditions... you just don't have time to get bored."

"How is driving my car like weight training?" she asked.

I explained. "If you're training correctly you can't be bored, just like driving. You're focused on your breathing, range of motion, form, cadence, rep number, mind/body connection. You most definitely don't have time to think about what you're having for brekky the next day!"

"Ok will you show me with a couple of sets?"

Totally impressed, I agreed, "You bet! Now you're talkin'. Let's rock!"

I didn't hear any snoring for the rest of our session.

Transferable Life Skill

Don't cruise through life ignoring the details. There will often be fine points that should not be ignored. Research your subject thoroughly to see if you're doing everything you can to achieve great results. Then do them to the best of your abilities.

PART 4

20% Recovery

This part of the fitness equation is REALLY overlooked by most people trying to transform their bodies and their lives. Research and real life results are showing that this factor is so critical that, NOT getting enough rest and recovery can thwart all the hard work you're doing in the playground and with your nutrition plan. Read on.

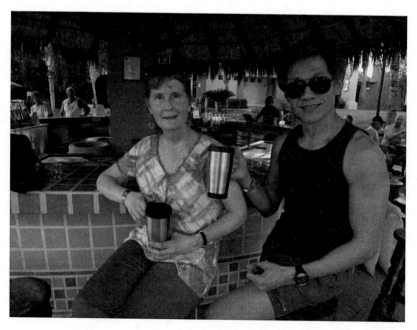

TheKim&I "decompressing" on our trip to PV!
Photo by Amanda Jean Malbeuf

CHAPTER 88

Ruth Anne's Story(Rest)

Do it NOW – sometimes "later" becomes "never"

After a particularly brutal body comp analysis, Ruth Anne was devastated. She worked so hard in the playground... level 10 intensity and tons of 'personal bests'. I certainly couldn't beat her up on her nutrition either. She had nailed the macronutrient ratios and caloric intake as close as anyone could expect. But she had lost a bit of valuable muscle and gained a pound of fat that week. Exactly opposite of the goal she worked so hard for.

"What happened?" she groaned.

"Hmmm, according to your nutrition log, you were almost spot on. So it wasn't that," I said, flipping through her food diary. "I was with you during each playground session so I know your training intensities and watched you achieve 'personal bests' in almost every session. Couldn't be that."

She was big time distraught. "Then what?"

"I'm going to say that it was lack of recovery time," I said.

A light bulb turned on. "I actually *have* been burning the midnight oil for the last few days," she said. "Right after work I was heading off to a temporary second job for a few hours each night."

"Recovery is one of the legs on a three legged stool," I said. "The first leg for transformation is to get micro tears in the muscle tissue from high intensity training. You're doing that. The second leg of the stool is to get enough amino acids from optimum protein sources to repair that tissue. According to your log, you're doing that. And if the third leg of the stool is not firmly on the ground, the stool falls over. That third leg is enough sleep to provide the recovery time to repair that tissue. You should be getting a minimum of seven hours of sleep each night, preferably more, to avoid the type of results that you got this week.

"Another way to think about it is, if you were flying a jet fighter on a long-distance critical mission, you know the plane can't stay in the air forever. Sooner or later it has to land, refuel and hit the hangar for maintenance and minor repairs. Same thing happens with your body. Recovery time is CRUCIAL!" I told her.

"Next week will be better," she said. "The second job was only for a week."

"And I know it will. In our Men's Groups, we would teach the 'Wheel of Life'. We would explain that your life is made up of aspects like Physical, Mental, Spiritual, Family, Social, Career, Recreation, and Financial components. We'd put each of them onto a pie chart representing spokes of a wheel. I would indicate to the men that if the spokes weren't balanced, the wheel would be wobbly and wouldn't turn very well, if at all. Then we had each man assess his own life to discover which spokes were too long or too short so that they could 'rebalance the wheel'. As you said, sometimes a spoke is too long for a short period of time, in your case, the career spoke. Other times a spoke needs an adjustment because it's causing the wheel to come to a dead stop."

Transferable Life Skill

Balance is the name of the game. If you neglect crucial aspects of any program you won't hit the target, or at the very least, it will take longer to achieve the goal, often at the expense of other areas of your life. In order to have a truly successful life, have a good hard look at each component and employ the "Rocking Chair Technique" : Sit yourself down in your rocking chair on your porch, 25 years down the road, and ask yourself what's important. Did you become one of the "Been Brothers" - "Coulda Been", "Woulda Been" or "Shoulda Been"? All related to "Aunt If Only"! It's not too late to change it in the "now".

CHAPTER 89

Rebecca's Story (Sleep)

Your power always belongs to you

"I haven't had a good sleep for months. I've just got way too much on my mind to get to sleep," Rebecca told me after our discussion about recovery. "Have you ever had sleep issues?" she asked.

"I tried a Fitbit for a while and it told me that I hit the pillow and I'm out within four to five minutes every time," I replied.

She stared at me in disbelief. "What? How?"

"I have a little technique I learned in 1975 and have used ever since... works every time."

"Care to share?" she begged.

"Ok. The trick as usual, is focus! First, lie down in the most comfy position that you can. Totally relax all of your muscles. Become a rag doll. Then take three HUGE breaths deep into your lungs and each time let the air out really, really slowly. Close your eyes. Then, and this is the crucial part that I find to be the most important component (because when I find myself straying from the technique, it will be right here) you must look up and back to the screen on the inside of your head."

"What? How do you do that?"

"With your eyes closed, look forward... then slowly roll your eyes up so that if you were to open your eyelids you're now looking up at your forehead. Then continue rolling your eyes back until you're looking at the back of your head. THIS is imperative. If I can't keep my eyes looking as far back as possible, I find the technique doesn't work and I have to refocus. Because when you lose focus, your eyes will naturally start looking forward again, and that's when you start thinking about what you're going to wear to work tomorrow. Happens every time."

"Ok, is that it?"

"Nope. Now, while you're looking at the screen in your mind, you have to visualize your toes. Wiggle them, move them in every direction, then totally relax them. Feel them become loose. Continue doing this with each muscle group as you work your way up to your head. I never make it past my thighs... ever."

"Wow, sounds like a lot of concentration."

"It is. It takes you away from your daily thoughts and into a relaxation state. I do it every night, and it works every night. Now, I do have another system for the times when I can cop a power nap during the day, but you have to really focus on this one as well."

"Yeah, let me try an easier one first," she said.

"Otay. While we're awake and conscious, our brains are usually in beta wave length, probably high beta if you're focusing on a problem. I know that for reparative sleep, my goal is to get into delta wave length as quickly as possible, or at least alpha. So as I again relax all my muscles and breathe deeply, I visualize the sine curve of the beta state. Then I tell myself to slow my mind, visualize the decreased sine frequency, leave the beta range and slowly move to mid beta, slow to low beta, alpha, theta, and then delta. I never make that one to alpha. I have great sleeps."

Transferable Life Skill

There are plenty of techniques for getting the job done. Don't discount any until you've tried them. Typically the more you focus on the strategy and the outcome you want, the better the results.

CHAPTER 90

Terry's Story (Hormones)
Neglect leads to more neglect

Terry was distressed. "Man, this whole transformation thing is taking longer than I thought. I'm putting ON pounds, not taking them off! I'm starting to lose sleep over this."

"Literally?" I asked.

"I've never slept well," he added.

I had just read an article on a website that morning so I shared it with him. "The Mayo Clinic published some research that I found very, very interesting. They said that if a person didn't sleep seven hours or more each night, that over a period of a year they would actually put on 17 pounds."

Terry was visibly shocked. "What? How could that be?"

"Apparently, when a person stays up late and gets less sleep, they're more tired the next day. So they don't tend to move as much and burn as many calories. Also, because they were up longer during the day, they had more time to eat more calories. Not a great combo!"

"Ok, that sorta makes sense."

He was open, so I added, "Then they mentioned the hormonal activity. More cortisol is released in the body to help with the extra stress of staying up later. Cortisol is a fat-storing, muscle-wasting hormone that causes cravings for sugar and carbohydrates to accommodate the fight or flight response.

"Also, your ghrelin and leptin get reversed. Ghrelin is a hormone that tells you it's time to chow down... go for it, pig out, find a buffet. Leptin tells you that you've had enough... time to stop filling your pie hole. So when they get reversed due to lack of sleep, the excess ghrelin courses through your system... you attack the refrigerator and stuff your face when you should be backing off. Then, again due to lack of sleep, leptin is in short supply and you can't stop shoveling truckloads of grease down your throat. Lack of recovery time is NOT your friend!"

Transferable Life Skill

Learn the repercussions of the technique you're using... or not using, and modify it according to what gets the results you're looking for. You must continue learning about new research that can explain why your results have been suffering. If you are not moving in the direction of your goal, a constant commitment to knowledge will more than likely hold the answer.

CHAPTER 91

JoLee's Story (Thyroid)
How hard will you work for what you want?

JoLee and her husband, Spiff, were next door neighbours who had just completed twelve weeks of the Body for Life program with me.

I could tell that JoLee wasn't exactly "ecstatic" about her results. She "only" lost 12 pounds and almost 10% body fat.

"What happened?" she groaned. "Why didn't I do better?"

"JoLee. First, let me say that there are a ton of folks out there who would kill to lose a pound a week, so congratulations on a great job.

"Now I was with you during each training session and I know how hard you worked, so that's not the issue. We got our micro tears.

"I was in my garage one day and watched you take a boat load of junk food out of your house to give away. I'm thinkin' you didn't take it out the back door to impress me, just to bring it back around and in the front door so that you could keep your stash. So I know you didn't sabotage yourself," I said. "You recorded your sleep and you typically got seven hours minimum every night. So all three legs of the stool were on the ground. There are a couple of other issues that we could consider but I think we should look at one in particular, and because you're a nurse, you might be able to fast track this one. Can you get a blood test to check your thyroid? If that little critter is acting up it can throw all your efforts out the window."

The following week, through her blood test, she discovered an under-active thyroid. Although it didn't make her feel better about the results of her program, it did open her eyes to an easily correctable health issue and explained her results.

Transferable Life Skill

Sometimes you can be doing everything right, or so you think. If you're not getting the results you want, dig deeper, analyze the situation further. There could be something important but not considered or unexpected that throws a wrench in to the works and derails your momentum.

CHAPTER 92

Naia's Story (Stretching)

The worst thing you can be is average

Naia waved to me from across the playground. As she walked toward me, I noticed an unusual angle in her neck. "Hey, I haven't seen you for a few weeks. How have you been doing?" I asked.

She moaned. "I just got back from a holiday in Mexico last night, which was great, but today I've got this stiff neck and shoulders. Do you ever get those little aches and pains?"

"Nothing that isn't self-inflicted," I replied.

I could hear her eyes roll. "Got a nice stretch for me?" she asked.

"Does Batman wear a cape? Try this. Put your hands behind your back. Grab your left wrist with your right hand. Now pull down gently with your right hand, and then tilt your head to your right shoulder as if you were listening to your shoulder. Get that nice stretch through the left side and then slowly turn your head so that you're now looking at that right shoulder. Ah, bliss!"

"Wow, it feels 100 percent better already!" she exclaimed after a few seconds.

"Now do the other side. This stretch works Pamfastically in the shower. Just add hot water!"

"I love this stretch, do you stretch regularly?" she asked.

"Naia, this is just between us girls, ok? Not to be shared with anyone!" I whispered.

"Ok." She leaned in close to me for the information.

"About ten years ago, Lexanne - you remember Lexanne, our supervisor at the time - told me that I was due for my annual recertification test and that she would role play a case study with me the following Saturday.

"Anyhoo, next Saturday rolls around and she got right into it by telling me that she's a 30 something mom of two who has been out of the playground since her first child was born, and she would like to lose some post baby fat and get into better shape so that she can pick up her kids with greater ease."

'Now take me through an appropriate program,' she says.

"After I asked her my usual questions about exercise history, meds, injuries, etc., I put her through a nice 're-intro' to the playground that balanced and covered all of her major muscle groups, and that wasn't too taxing on her first time out.

"At the end of the session Lexanne started adding up all the points on the clip board that she was carrying, to mark my performance.

"'Well,' she said. 'I was going to give you 100 percent, but I can't.'

I stared at her and said, "Whatchoo talkin' bout?"

She said that I did a perfect program but I didn't get her to stretch!

"So I would have received a perfect score if I had you stretch?" I asked her.

'Yep, sorry.'

"Ok," I said. "But can I just say three things about that?"

"Sure."

So I went for it. "First, stretching as a warm up, is quite controversial. Some research shows that it does absolutely nothing, and some shows that it can actually be a detriment. So really, it should be an individual choice.

"Second, the ONLY time I have EVER stretched in over 60 years is to relieve a cramp, and I'm doing pretty good.

"And third, I DO take all of my new members to the chart in the stretching area and tell them that, should they want to stretch, all the instructions are right there on the wall. They really don't need me to show them how to do it. What they need me to do is to coach proper range of motion, breathing, form and mind/body connection... way more important!

"Lexanne smiled and said, '100 percent, now get outta here!'"

Naia responded. "Well I like to stretch, so thanks for the great story. Gotta go stretch now! See ya."

Transferable Life Skill

Some "conventional knowledge" is only "common practice" and some "practices" are superfluous and can be eliminated from the equation when unnecessary. Test drive methods to determine if they, in fact, are beneficial for YOU and if they are really necessary.

CHAPTER 93

Bert's Story (Delegate)

It's time to parent yourself

After I explained how important his health and fitness were to him, and how he needed to establish exercise as a top priority, for himself AND his young son, Bert berated me. "I'm a single dad and I have a really demanding job. I have too many things to do to fit exercise into my routine on a regular basis!"

"Bert," I said. "Sorry to upset you like this but can I share something with you that not many people know about me?"

"Please do."

I continued. "Make no mistake please. I'm not dissing you or belittling you in any way. Knowing you, I'm absolutely certain that you're doing the best job you can possibly do right now in a rather tough situation.

"In fact, we share a lot in common. I was also a single parent for over 15 years to my beautiful little daughter. Plus I was a partner in a very busy company. Not only that but, at that time, my ego told me that 'ONLY I' could do the job correctly and efficiently. I was running myself ragged... UNTIL, I learned to let some things go. I could delegate certain jobs and it would open up more time for the more important priorities in my life.

"Bert, take a step back and sincerely ask yourself if there is any way, any way at all, that you can delegate something, anything, that can loosen up valuable time that you could be spending on your health. I know you'll always do the job better than someone else but they will, in time, learn how to do it satisfactorily."

"You're right," he said. "There are a couple of things I can think of right now that I could hand off to someone else. And I know I'll feel better all day if I can do my work out every morning!"

"Now you're talkin'. THAT's the right attitude! Possibility thinking at it's very best! U Rock!" I said.

Bert was more consistent in the playground than ever after our little chat.

Transferable Life Skill

Control can be a "balance issue". There may be times when it's wise to relinquish some control in order to reap the more valuable reward. If you're stressed out and contemplating your priorities, consider this technique: Automate... Delegate... or Eliminate! A task deleted is a task completed!

PART 5

The Plan Man!

I wasn't going to include an exercise plan in this book, and I'm still not going to, because there are waaaaaay too many exercise books and websites out there. Each one is very helpful in its own way but really, if a person needs an exercise program your friendly neighbourhood trainer is more than willing to help out or at the very least, Google is your friend.

Having said that, what is 30/30/20/20 if I leave out one of the 20's? So I decided that as a trainer with 45 years of experience in the playground, I should provide you with what I consider to be THE most effective transformation exercises for each major muscle group that I have seen and experienced. These are the ones that I use for the transformation portion of my own annual four part periodization program (see Chapter 82).

Please keep in mind that this program is not for bodybuilders. This is for the average person who wants to change their body composition, namely to lose body fat and build a reasonable amount of muscle.

All of these exercises must be done with barbells and dumbbells.

Why not at home with body weight exercises you ask?

Funny you should ask. Because you will be doing body weight exercises until the proverbial cows come home. That's why. Think push-ups. A person who wants optimal transformation results will eventually be able to lift more than their body weight in a chest press but if they do push-ups to achieve a mediocre result, they would be doing them all day.

As I said, there are tons of exercise books out there, along with Google and Youtube, so I will not dwell on how to do the exercises or the proper form. Instead I will provide the all-time best exercises that I've discovered over the years in the order that you should apply them. These are progressive exercises, meaning that you need to start with light resistance and work up. There are lots of fancy dancy exercises and variations but these are the BASIC BEST ones to get the job done!

I will count on the fact that you didn't skip reading the book and go straight to this section. Because if you did, you're gonna be disappointed and have a bunch of questions. Go back and read the rest of the book and stop trying to shortcut the process (this is yet another transferable life skill)!

Otay, here goes:

Barbell squats - aim for at least a ninety degree range of motion to fire the glutes. Start with half your body weight. Yeah that's right... half! You're going to be doing over your body weight so you may as well start here. Why delay the inevitable?

Dumbbell lunges - "Everybody Loves Raymond" but nobody loves lunges

Deadlifts – again work up to body weight

3 Position Barbell Calf Raises - skis, ducks and pigeons

Dumbbell Flat Bench Press - this is where the "kick up" is your best friend (see Chapter 75 – TheKim's Story).

Pull Ups - best exercise for the back in... ever! If you can't do them... again... go back and read the book (Chapter 11 – Daphne's Story)!

Dumbbell Shoulder Press - I was going to choose side laterals but it's easier to maintain proper form and range of motion with this one. Plus the big bonus is that you could end up doing hand stand push-ups! So kewl!

Dips - again skull crushers are a "go to" exercise, but can be tricky and a bit dangerous (hence the name). This exercise is much more progressable.

Incline Dumbbell Bicep Curl - a classic... the Gun Show!

Killer Abs – go to nowgogetpumped.com

PART 6

Conclusion

Now as I said in the intro, we can change the world to be a much better place. People are hurting. People are stuck. They're aching for accomplishment, fulfillment, purpose and joy! In my career I have seen incredible changes in people who have transformed themselves to have their best bodies ever. They come to realize that the journey was not really a physical one, although it WAS physically demanding. They realize that it was really a mental odyssey... laughing... crying... advancing... retreating... disappointment... euphoria... but overall... extremely rewarding, and learning really great lessons in a life-long journey that will pay huge dividends all the days of their lives. They have become physically, mentally, nutritionally, and functionally healthy.

Once you realize that you can transfer and incorporate all the skills you learned in this book to every aspect of your life, you will find success is indeed possible.

But now it's time to pay it forward... DO NOT forget our deal! It's time to help two people who have witnessed your transformation and shown interest in replicating your success. It's time to help them achieve the same success. It's time to help them transfer the skills to *their* lives. Help them feel fulfilled. It's time to change the planet! I sincerely thank you for your contribution and for joining our team!

nowgogetpumped!!!

PART 7

Two Thumbs Up from
Clients and Members

"Who makes up these stupid exercises anyway?"
– Doc Miller (as he was attempting to do a new exercise)

"Are you kidding?"
– Jan (after my request for one more rep)

"You have a lot of talents Randy, but counting is not one of them!"
– Roxanne

"I love doing my Dips 'n' Doodles!"
– Gio (after I told him that dips were next up)

"Randy... I have a love/hate relationship with you!"
– Christy

"THIS... was a mistake!"
– Doc Miller (as he was performing a Bosu Arnie Press)

"If you eat it, write it!"
– Yanny

"He said put it into turbo boost... not turtle boost!"
– Bryce

"Thirteen! Just managing expectations!"

– Doc Miller (When I requested his intensity level on the last rep of his Bosu step over. He knew thatwe had to raise the weight if the intensitywasn't high enough.)

"Oops, I shouldn't have done that!"

– Ann (just after I caught her rolling her eyes when she discovered the weights were too light)

"I'd rather have the odd little ache from working out than the constant aches and pains from getting old!"

– Christy

"I like the TRX way better than the whirligig!" (Lebert SRT bar)

– Jan

"Oh dear! I've got work to do!"

– Drew (when he couldn't complete his final dip rep)

PART 8

Bonus Bumpa Stickers

My beautiful little granddaughter, Amanda, couldn't say "Grandpa" when she was just learning to talk so she called me "Bumpa". Believe me when I say that I have been called a lot of names in my time, but I love this one. And it's stuck to this day (she's now 25 years old), and all my family and closest friends call me by this name!

So as a huge bonus to motivate and inspire you... I share with you, my "Bumpa Stickers". Read each one. Stop at the first one that resonates with you. Internalize and use it for the day. Don't read the rest until the next day and repeat.

For more Bumpa Stickers go to nowgogetpumped.com

BUMPA STICKERS

One life... one body... no excuses!

Don't stand around on the outside of life looking in, get in the middle and squeeze the juice out of it!

You don't want to need help getting off a toilet seat when you're eighty!

Believe you can and you're half way there!

If not now... when?

Don't live to eat, eat to live!

I'd rather miss a meal than miss my work out!

I CAN because I think I CAN!

Confidence is the key to everything; it's also the key to everything!

Your results will always be in direct proportion to your effort!

You don't want to be on the lower end of the fitness continuum!

Attitude is EVERYTHING!

You have all the time there is, nobody has more time than you do, so it's time to work out!

Are you fit enough to survive?

Discipline is doing what needs to be done... even if you don't want to!

Be the one who didn't give up on their dream!

Doubt kills more dreams than failure ever will!

A year from now you'll wish you had started today!

Push yourself because nobody's going to do it for you!

How bad do you want it?

I prefer the pain of discipline over the pain of regret!

Excuses don't burn calories!

Don't just wish for a great body... WORK FOR IT!

Don't be upset by the results you didn't get from the workout you didn't do!

If it were easy, everybody would be doing it and everybody would look like a fitness model!

Don't stop when you're tired, stop when you're done!

Let's DO this!

If others can do this, so can I!

How do you eat an elephant – one bite at a time!

Giving up is NOT an option!

The fitter you are - the better you feel!

The only place "success" comes before "sweat" is in the dictionary!

You never fail until you quit trying!

Minimum efforts give minimum results, maximum efforts give maximum results!

If you want something you've never had, you have to do something you've never done!

nowgogetpumped!!!

Gratitudes

My long time personal clients (many who have become very close friends) have been a huge motivation to write this book. I very graciously thank every one of them for their loyalty, friendship and support. In particular, Dr. J.C. Mullen and wife Yannick, Judge Rosanna Saccomani Q.C. and hubby Ian, Tema Frank and hubby Dr. J.M. Shaw, Dr. J. Esaw, Dr. T. Orsten and wife Chris, Teresa Haykowsky and hubby Tom, Dr. G. Frank and wife Rheva, Deb Miller Q.C., Dr. B. Allenby and wife Didi, Dr. T. Verco, Dr. L. Wincott and wife Karen, JoAnn Creore, Heidi Paranych, Abel Shiferaw, Gil Heise, Stuart Mackay & wife Judy, and Lois Browne.

A huge shout out to the staff and members of the Edmonton YMCA, who have provided me with over twenty years of fun and precious learning opportunities, especially Kent Bittorf, Asim Chin, Taylor Cheung, Zachary Lun, Julianna Wickins, Jennifer Bustamante, Jenna Buckley, Tara Mayne, Heather Scherer, and Edie Dixon.

Great appreciation goes to Canfitpro for all the fantastic events and certification courses where I have learned so much.

I would like to thank Bob Proctor for creating the dream and for his kind encouraging words way back in 1975 at his incredible life changing XOCES seminar in Red Deer, Alberta.

I owe a huge debt of gratitude to my master mind group, Claudia Sammer - strategist extraordinaire, Shoma Sinha – gifted business pro, Tema Frank – writing consultant/marketing/production adviser splendida, Al Tejani – website/tech/marketing guru, Ajay Bhardwaj - communications wizard/writing consultant, JoAnn Creore – writing consultant/superfit senior, Jon Hall – publishing/marketing advisor, Will Leddy – thought master, Ernest Augustus – photographer, Ju

Zhang – "The Chinese Connection" liaison, and Gordon Hearn - liaison.

Also, big bouquets go to our beautiful granddaughter Amanda Jean Malbeuf.

And as always, my FUNtabulous and ABSolutely wonderful wife, Kim... for her unyielding faith in me and all of her encouragement, love and devotion... the All-Time Best promoter on the planet! But it's her precious giving heart that has inspired me to realize my dream of helping people to realize their own. I wanna be just like her when I grow up!

About the Author

Randy is a busy chronologically enhanced senior (67 years young) certified personal fitness and lifestyle trainer, who lives in Edmonton, Alberta, Canada with his wife Kim. He is a Canfitpro PTS, NWL, Certified TRX Suspension Trainer and YMCA Certified Strength and Conditioning Leader, with a background in Psychology.

He was a national fitness club manager at the age of 21, and later became a motivational speaker and consultant with Success Motivation Institute. He has been the recipient of the PAAFE Man of Honour Award and was the YMCA Bill Reese Volunteer of the Year.

He is available for speaking engagements, consultation or training and can be reached at nowgogetpumped.com

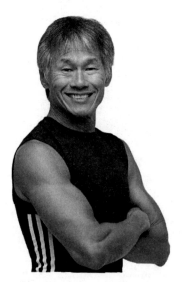

Photo by Ernest Augustus